Second Edition

Food and Nutritional Science

with OBJECTIVE QUESTIONS and ANSWERS

Text for students of health and home sciences
and
Guide for those appearing in competitive examinations

W0225626

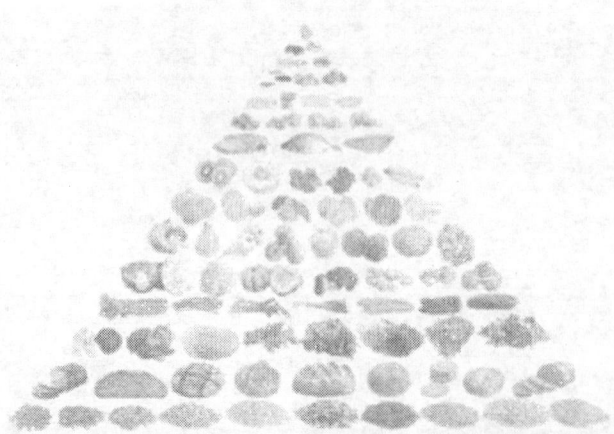

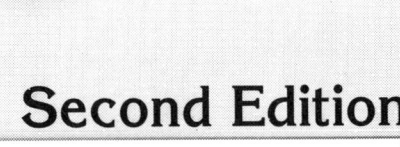

Second Edition

Food and Nutritional Science

with OBJECTIVE QUESTIONS and ANSWERS

Text
and
Guide

for students of health and home sciences

for those appearing in competitive examinations

Pooja Verma
MSc (Nutrition), BEd, UGC-NET/JRF, PhD Scholar

Department of Human Development and Family Studies
School for Home Sciences
Babasaheb Bhimrao Ambedkar University
(Central University)
Lucknow, UP

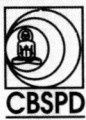

CBSPD

CBS Publishers & Distributors Pvt Ltd

New Delhi • Bengaluru • Chennai • Kochi • Kolkata • Lucknow • Mumbai
Hyderabad • Jharkhand • Nagpur • Patna • Pune • Uttarakhand

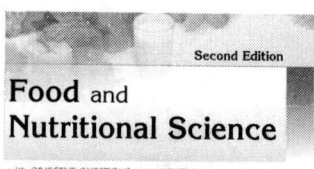

Second Edition

Food and Nutritional Science

with OBJECTIVE QUESTIONS and ANSWERS

ISBN: 978-93-87964-08-2

Copyright © Author and Publisher

Second Edition: 2021
Reprint: 2024
First Edition: 2016

Published by **Satish Kumar Jain** and produced by **Varun Jain** for

CBS Publishers & Distributors Pvt Ltd
4819/XI Prahlad Street, 24 Ansari Road, Daryaganj, New Delhi 110 002, India.
Ph: 011-23289259, 23266861
Website: www.cbspd.com
e-mail: delhi@cbspd.com

Corporate Office: 204 FIE, Industrial Area, Patparganj, Delhi 110 092
Ph: 011-4934 4934
Fax: 011-4934 4935   e-mail: publishing@cbspd.com;publicity@cbspd.com

Branches

- **Bengaluru:** Seema House 2975, 17th Cross, K.R. Road, Banasankari 2nd Stage, Bengaluru 560 070, Karnataka, India
  Ph: +91-80-26771678/79   Fax: +91-80-26771680   e-mail: bangalore@cbspd.com
- **Chennai:** 7, Subbaraya Street, Shenoy Nagar, Chennai 600 030, Tamil Nadu, India
  Ph: +91-44-26680620, 26681266   Fax: +91-44-42032115   e-mail: chennai@cbspd.com
- **Kochi:** 42/1325, 1326, Power House Road, Opp KSEB, Ernakulam 682 018, Kochi, Kerala, India
  Ph: +91-484-4059061-67   Fax: +91-484-4059065   e-mail: kochi@cbspd.com
- **Kolkata:** 147, Hind Ceramics Compound, 1st Floor, Nilgunj Road, Belghoria, Kolkata 700 056, West Bengal, India
  Ph: +91-33-25633055/56   e-mail: kolkata@cbspd.com
- **Lucknow:** Basement, Khushnuma Complex, 7-Meerabai Marg (Behind Jawahar Bhawan), Lucknow 226 001, UP, India
  Ph: +0552-4000032   e-mail:tiwari.lucknowi@cbspd.com
- **Mumbai:** PWD Shed. Gala no. 25/26, Ramchandra Bhatt Marg, Next to JJ Hospital Gate no. 2, Opp. Union Bank of India, Noorbaug, Mumbai 400 009, Maharashtra, India
  Ph: 022-66661880/89   e-mail: mumbai@cbspd.com

Representatives

| • Hyderabad | 0-9885175004 | • Jharkhand | 0-9811541605 | • Nagpur | 0-8692091830 |
| • Patna | 0-9334159340 | • Pune | 0-9664372571 | • Uttarakhand | 0-9716462459 |

Printed at: Rashtriya Printers, Dilshad Garden, Delhi, India

to

my loving mother
Smt Geeta Verma

Preface to the Second Edition

It gives me immense pleasure to present the new edition of *Food and Nutritional Science with Objective Questions*. The new edition focuses on the recent advances and the novel approaches in the field of food and nutritional science. The book presents the latest information about the concepts of food and nutritional science and highlights that how technology is applied in food preparation and formulations of new food products. The microbial deterioration of foods and how food can be prevented from microbial spoilage are well explained. The new edition of book deals with the nutritional benefits of food and how food acts as medicine.

The book serves as an ideal for the students who are studying home science, food and nutrition, food science and technology, agriculture, and allied areas. The contents in this edition have been revised on the basis of recent developments in the field of food and nutritional science along with the changes in the competitive exams.

In the new edition the following six chapters have been added:
- Food and Nutrition Trends: 2020 (Chapter 2)
- Basic of Nutrition (Chapter 3)
- Food Microbiology (Chapter 9)
- Food Waste and its Management (Chapter 10)
- Applications of Nanotechnology in Nutrition (Chapter 11)
- Nutraceuticals (Chapter 12)

As in the earlier edition, there were 1000 objective questions but in the new edition 1500 objective questions have been given to help the students who are preparing for various competitive exams. The terminologies used in the chapters are explained and are included in the glossary at the end of the book.

I hope that the new edition helps the students in understanding the concepts and importance of nutrition and helps in learning the novel techniques in combating the problems of health and nutritional disorders.

I am grateful to the staff of CBS Publishers & Distributors Pvt Ltd, New Delhi, for their contribution in the completion of the new edition of book.

Pooja Verma

Preface to the First Edition

Food and nutritional science is one of the growing fields of science in the present time. It is now leading towards the new path which involves the new innovations and applications in the sector of food production. New trends in food processing and preservation techniques have been developed which are moving forward for combating the problems of hunger and malnutrition.

The concept of food and nutrition science in the recent years have adopted various new trends which are not only satisfying the hunger needs but also helping in curing the diseases, which develops due to unhealthy lifestyle. Due to change in the dietary behavior today, the dietitians and food technologists are trying to modify and develop the food items for meeting the needs of the nutrition.

One of the major goals of today is to improve the nutritional quality of food and to make food more healthy and nutritious. The technologists and scientists are exploring the nature and developing food items which are not only healthy but also curative. The skills and techniques applied in the food research are aimed at increasing food production and making food nutritious.

The other problem faced by many people today is the lifestyle disorders. These disorders occur due to the unhealthy food practices and lack of knowledge about the nutritional attributes of food items. Food and nutritional science is an emerging field which guides and helps in understanding the food and nutrition and its related issues. This knowledge will help in understanding the nutritional aspects of food so that the diet is modified for preventing the disease.

This book contains the knowledge of food science and technology and other nutrition-related concepts. This book also contains 1000 objective type questions which will help the students in learning about food and nutrition. The book will serve as an ideal text for students and help them develop confidence, especially those who are preparing for various competitive examinations.

I would like to thank my professors who have directly or indirectly helped me in writing this book. My sincere thanks to my friends who have enabled me to write this book. My special thanks to my parents who helped me and guide me at each and every step during the compilation of this book.

I truly hope that the readers and the students appearing in competitive examinations will enjoy this book. Suggestions and comments are welcome for future editions.

Pooja Verma

Contents

Food Science and Technology

India has always attracted other nations due to its huge treasure of natural reserves specially food items. The vast store of grains, fruits, vegetables and oilseeds have made in India, a well developed country and has helped in raising its economy. This is the reason that is why India holds good relations with other country especially in the field of exporting. Recent advancements in the area of food production and development are now reducing the burden of exporting food items and this is only made possible due to the use of recent technology in the area of food production. Rapid industrialization and increase in the population have pushed the technologists and scientists who work in the field of food, to produce, to modify or to extract something from the natural food items which could help the people in spending less time in kitchen or at home, making the things easy and spending less time in preparation and cooking of food. This all have become possible only due to food technology.

Food technology is a branch of food science that deals with the production processes that make foods. Early scientific research into food technology concentrated on food preservation.

It is also defined as the technology in which food science is applied in manufacturing and preservation of food products. The food technologists study the chemical, physical and microbiological makeup of the food. The food is processed, preserved, packaged and stored according to the specifications laws and standards set up by industry and government.

Food science is the discipline in which biology, physical sciences, and engineering are used to study the nature of foods, the causes of their deterioration, and the principles underlying food processing are also studied.

Food technology is the application of food science to the selection, preservation, processing, packaging, distribution, and use of safe, nutritious, and wholesome food.

Food science is the study of the physical, biological, and chemical makeup of food; the causes of food deterioration; and the concepts underlying food.

Food scientists and technologists apply scientific disciplines including chemistry, engineering, microbiology, and nutrition to the study of food to improve the safety, nutrition, wholesomeness and availability of food.

Food scientists may develop ways to process, preserve, package, and/or store food according to industry and government specifications and regulations.

Food Technology also Involves

- The selection, preservation, processing, packaging, distribution, and use of safe food.
- Related fields include:
  - *Analytical food chemistry*
  - *Biotechnology*
  - *Food engineering*
  - *Nutrition*
  - *Quality control*
  - *Food safety management*

Food Processing and Manufacturing

- Food processing is one of the valuable sector in India.
- Food processing is the treatment of food substances by changing their properties to preserve it, improve its quality or make it functionally more useful.
- Food processors take raw fruits, vegetables, or marine foods and transform them into edible products through the application of technical aspects and scientific knowledge.
- Chemical, biological, and mechanical processes are used to convert relatively bulky, perishable, and typically inedible food materials into shelf-stable, convenient, and palatable foods and beverages.
- According to the Food and Drug Administration (FDA), there are approximately 44,000 food processors and 1,13000 food warehouses in the US that provide processed foods to our country, and exports throughout the world. The processors include canners, producers, wineries, and other food and beverage manufacturers and distributors.
- There are more than 1.2 million retail food facilities (restaurants, grocery stores, and others) that serve or sell foods directly to consumers.

Food Manufacturing

Food manufacturing is the mass production of food products from raw animal and plant materials, using principles of food technology.

Food Research

Food research is the careful, systematic study, investigation, and compilation of information about foods and their components.

Product Development

Product development is the innovative aspect in food product industry, it involves creation of new flavors, colors or varieties of existing products and/or the creation of entirely new products. This also involves enhancing the nutritional qualities of food by applying scientific principles and incorporation of their nutritive food items.

Quality Assurance and Quality Control

Both quality assurance and quality control involve the process of ensuring that products are manufactured correctly and that ingredients and finished products are tested and meet safety and quality specifications.

Food Regulation

Food regulation is safety aspect in food product industry. It is the process of determining standards for products, defining safety, and inspecting products. Regulations are set by governments.

Food Biotechnology and Genetically Modified Foods

According to Oxford dictionary: *Biotechnology involves the genetic manipulation of the microorganisms for the production of antibiotics, hormones, etc.*

In the area of food research biotechnology is applied for the qualitative and quantitative production of foods. Biotechnology involves the principle of genetic engineering that is the genetic material called deoxyribonucleic acid (DNA) is transferred from a cell of one species to another unrelated species to express itself in the recipient cells. This is also known as recombinant DNA technology. Foods modified through the transfer of genes are known as genetically modified foods (GM foods).

Biotechnology involves various disciplines such as microbiology, chemical engineering, fermentation technology, genetics and enzymatic properties. The tasks of biotechnology are complicated but they have various benefits. Food prepared by this process is called genetically modified food (GM food). The GM foods are cheaper and are nutritious and healthy. These foods are playing important role in preventing hunger and malnutrition. Iron-rich rice, quality protein maize, high carotene-sweet potato and micronutrient rich seeds are some of the outcomes of research in food biotechnology.

Role of Food Technology in Research and Development

The research and development in food technology has resulted into the production of safe and nutritious foods. The food processing industries manufacture a large variety of food products. They include the primary foods like rice and wheat products, oil, sugar and pulses. They are processed to convert into edible form.

Food technology courses can be a good career option. There is increasing scope of food technology courses in India.

Scope of Food Technology Courses in India

Today, several career opportunities are available in India. One can opt for various food technology courses for a bright career. Food processing industry is rapidly growing in India and several employment opportunities are available in various industries. There is good scope of food technology courses which offer numerous job opportunities in various areas.

People can get jobs in food processing industries, research laboratories, hotels, soft drink factories, quality control, rice mills, manufacturing industries and distilleries.

In India, food processing industry is accelerating fast as the consumer food industry, which includes pasta, breads, cakes, pastries, corn flakes, ready to eat and ready to cook products, cocoa products, biscuits, soft drinks, beer, alcohol beverages, mineral and packaged water and segment of consumer foods is seeing an upward trend.

The Cabinet of India on June 21, 2007, granted its approval to an integrated plan, which aims to promote India's food processing sector and boost the country's agricultural business (according to a press release). As per the report there are about 300 million upper- and middle-class consumers of processed and packaged food in the country, and another 200 million are likely to be added by 2010.

There is another concept arising is the development of food parks. Ministry of Food Processing Industries is planning to establish 500 food parks in the Tenth Five-Year Plan across every parliamentary constituency. This will give a further boost to the growth and development of food processing industries and thereby is generating a huge job potential for those who have an aptitude for the work and required qualifications. The food processing industry is still at its growing stage in India. It thus provides ample employment opportunities.

The areas where one can find employment in this industry are

- Food processing companies
- Food research laboratories

- Food wholesalers
- Food inspector
- Food analysts
- Retailers
- Restaurants provide employment to candidates with degrees in home science and specializations in food technology, nutrition or food services management. Diploma holders in dietetics, applied nutrition, food science and preservation and those having certificate in dietetics or food and nutrition can also be employed in this industry.
- Bacteriologist, toxicologists and those trained in packaging technology, organic chemistry, biochemistry and analytical chemistry can find opening food technology laboratories or in quality control departments.
- A number of public sector undertakings in the department of food also require people in this field. The Food Corporation of India, which handles the purchase, storage transport and distribution of food grains and other food items, provide employment to large number of people. Modern Food Corporation which markets bread, fruit juices, edible oils, soft drink concentrates and North-Eastern Agricultural Marketing Corporation which markets and process fruits and vegetables also recruits people.
- Self-employment opportunities also exist in the form of dynamic delivery networks for those who want to work on their own.
- Private sector companies have been the key players in the food sector companies are now moving into the sector, seeing the potential in processed foods.

Some other scopes are

- Bakers
- Meat, poultry, trimmers, and fish cutters
- Slaughterers and meat packers
- Food batch makers

- Food cooking machine operators and tenders
- Food and tobacco roasting, baking and drying machine operators and tenders.

In India, the major industries of private sector are

- Godrej industries Limited
- Nestle India Pvt. Ltd.
- Britannia Industries Ltd.
- Hindustan Lever Limited
- Milk food
- ITC Limited
- Parle Products Pvt. Ltd.
- Agro Tech Foods
- Amul
- Perfetti India Ltd.
- Cadbury India Ltd.
- PepsiCo India Holdings
- Gits Food Products Pvt. Ltd.
- Dabur India Ltd.

Nature of Work

Food technologists, technicians, biotechnologists and engineers are required in this industry for the practical application of the principles of many disciplines of science in the manufacturing or production, preservation and packaging, processing and canning of various food products. All this needs preparation of raw materials for processing which involves selection, or cleaning of the raw material, followed by the actual processing, which could be chopping, blanching, crushing, mixing or even cooking of the food item, the addition of preservatives and the final packaging along with keep in hygiene ... maintaining quality of products.

People Working in Food Processing Industry

Food technologists: They are given the responsibility of determining whether a particular process is being performed in a certain specified way or not. They are instrumental in devising new ways and improving the older ones for preserving, conserving and processing food. They have to check for the contamination, adulteration and controlling the nutritional value of the food products which are to be processed. Food technologists are also assigned to determine to quality of the raw materials used in the food which has to be dispatched to the market. They also look after the storage conditions and hygiene.

FERMENTATION

Fermentation is one of the most important food processing technologies. Many fermented products are preserved with extension of shelf life. In addition to being more shelfstable products and removal of antinutritional components, all fermented foods have aroma and flower characteristics that result directly or indirectly from the fermenting microorganisms. The most common groups of microorganisms involved in food fermentation are bacteria, yeasts, and molds. Microbial enzymes also play an important role in food fermentation. Fermented foods play an important role in improving food security, increasing income and employment, enhancing livelihoods and improving the nutrition and social wellbeing of millions of people around the world, and others. A fermentation is influenced by numerous factors, including moisture, temperature, dissolved O_2 concentration, and dissolved CO_2. Variation of these factors may affect the rate of fermentation, the organoleptic properties of the product, nutritional quality, and other physicochemical properties. Fermentation preserves perishable raw materials.

Types of Fermentation

There are three types of fermentation

- **Lactic acid fermentation:** In the lactic acid fermentation, yeast strains and bacteria convert starches or sugars into lactic acid. There is not any requirement of heat in preparation. Foods such as sauerkraut, pickles, yoghurt and sour dough bread are the examples.
- **Ethanol/alcohol fermentation:** Where the pyruvate molecules in starches or sugars are broken down by yeasts into alcohol and carbon dioxide molecules to produce wine and beer.
- **Acetic acid fermentation:** In acetic acid fermentation, involves fermentation of starches or sugars from grains or fruit into sour tasting vinegar and condiments. This is the difference, for example, between apple cider vinegar and apple cider.

Health benefits of fermented foods

Fermented foods are very healthy and have good nutritional value. These foods contain healthy live bacteria known as probiotics and fermented foods that have gone through a process during which bacteria converts the starches and sugars in that food into lactic acid and acetic acid.

These foods contain nutrients such as vitamin K_2, trace minerals, B-vitamins and probiotics. The other advantages are: They are easy to prepare and economical. Fermentation is an old food preservation method and was used in many forms such as sauerkraut, lassi— a yogurt drink, fermented milk, some pickles such as cabbage, turnips, eggplant, cucumbers, onions, squash, and carrots and yoghurt.

Some other health benefits are

- Improves digestion.
- Keeps immune system strong.
- Improves mood and behavior.
- Helps in preventing lifestyle diseases.
- The beneficial bacteria present in fermented foods are detoxifiers, capable of drawing out a wide range of toxins and heavy metals from the body.

ENCAPSULATION

Encapsulation involves the incorporation of food ingredients, enzymes, cells or other materials in small capsules. In food industry, the applications have increased because of the fact that encapsulated materials can be protected from moisture, heat or other extreme conditions, thus enhancing their stability and maintaining viability. Encapsulation in foods is also utilized to mask odours or tastes. Various techniques are employed to form the capsules, including spray drying, spray chilling or spray cooling, extrusion coating, fluidized bed coating, liposome entrapment, coacervation, inclusion complexation, centrifugal extrusion and rotational suspension separation. Each of these techniques is discussed in this review.

Examples of food items

- Flavouring agents, acids bases, artificial sweeteners, colourants, preservatives, leavening agents, antioxidants, agents with undesirable flavours, odours and nutrients, among others.
- The use of encapsulation for sweeteners such as aspartame and flavours in chewing gum is well known.
- Fats, starches, dextrins, alginates, protein and lipid materials can be employed as encapsulating materials.
- The addition of water to dry beverages or cake mixes is an example.
- Liposomes have been applied in cheese-making, and its use in the preparation of food emulsions such as spreads, margarine and mayonnaise is a developing area.
- Most recent developments include the encapsulation of foods in the areas of controlled release, carrier materials, preparation methods and sweetener immobilization.

EXTRACTION

Extraction is an example of a separation technique and is used in several food industries. It can split two components, separate them apart. The extraction can be from solid to liquid, liquid to liquid and so on. The technique of extraction involves movement of one or more compounds of interest (analytes) from one phase or their original location (usually referred as the sample or matrix) to another phase or physically separated location where further processing and analysis occurs. The use of a convenient type of extraction not only influences the accuracy of the results but also determines the total analysis time and in this way affects the sample and the analysis. The extraction process can be categorized into two classes: Conventional and advanced techniques. The conventional technique of extraction requires longer time and larger amounts of solvent. To overcome these problems, some advanced techniques have been designed. These include ultrasound assisted extraction, microwave assisted extraction, high pressure extraction (HPE), and addition of cosolvents.

ENZYME TECHNOLOGY

Enzyme is a kind of catalytically active protein. In the past, the enzyme used in food processing was mostly derived from animal and plant extracts. Most of the enzymes used are now from microbial fermentation. In general, the purity of the enzyme used in food processing does not need to be particularly high, mostly partially purified enzyme. Most enzymes applied in the food processing are glucoamylase and then followed by protease, lipase, esterase, oxidoreductase and isomerase.

Flour product

Enzymes play a significant role in a variety of special flour production and transformation. For example, in improving the baking quality, nutritional quality, texture, storage resistance and other function of flour products.

The major enzymes used for flour modification are listed in the table below.

Dairy industry: The important enzymes used in dairy processing are catalase and lactase. Lactase can reduce the content of lactose to produce low lactose milk, low lactose hydrolyzed milk can improve the milk flavor, sweetness and nutritional value. In fermented milk, the use of lactase can accelerate the reaction and improve the fermentation efficiency to make fermented milk unique

frankincense flavor and relatively extend shelf life of the product.

Meat products processing: Enzyme used in the meat industry is mainly used to improve product quality (color, smell, taste, etc.) and increase the added value of by-products.

Fruit and vegetable industry: Enzymes used in this area are mainly pectin, cellulase and amylase, and mostly are used alone or in combination. These enzymes are mainly used for peeling fruit, clarifying fruit juice, reducing the viscosity of fruit juice, increasing the rate of fruit juices, enhance stability, what's more, they are also applied in making vegetable juice, extending the shelf life of fruits and vegetables, reducing nutrient loss and so on.

Major enzymes used for flour modification

Enzyme name	Function
α-amylase	• Make bread volume increased
	• Loose texture
	• Dough fermentation
	• Improve the bread structure
	• Good and stable bread color
	• Improve the furnace into the swelling; anti-aging
	• Improve bread elasticity and taste
Glucose oxidase	• Prolong the stabilization time
	• Reduce the softening degree
	• Improve the tensile and gelatinization characteristics of the flour
	• Increase the tensile resistance
	• Increasing the bread size
	• Improve the noodles bite taste
Protease	• Weakening the gluten to soften the dough to improve the viscoelasticity
	• Shortening the mixing time of the dough, improving the baking quality
	• Making the product easy to shape
	• Improves the taste.
Lipase	• Delaying the aging of starch
	• Increasing the stability of dough fermentation
	• Increasing the volume of bread and improving the bread quality and preservation ability
	• Reducing the spots on the dough, increasing the bite force, making the noodles not sticking in the boiled water, not easy to break

Beverage industry: Enzymes are also used in deep processing of tea. Enzyme tannase can improve the tea cold-soluble, prevent tea cloudy, and can improve the strength of the strength of tea.

BIOTECHNOLOGY IN FOOD INDUSTRY

Biotechnology = bios (life) + techno (tools) + logos (study of). Biotechnology as a science deals with the applicability of various living organisms in development of useful products.

Food biotechnology is the application of modern biotechnological techniques to the manufacture and processing of food. Fermentation of food, which is the oldest biotechnological process, and food additives, as well as plant and animal cell cultures, are included. New developments in fermentation and enzyme technological processes, genetic engineering, protein engineering, bioengineering, and processes involving monoclonal antibodies have introduced exciting dimensions to food biotechnology. Although traditional agriculture and crop breeding are not generally regarded as food biotechnology, agricultural biotechnology, i.e., of animal and plant foods, is expected to become an increasingly important "engine" of development for the agri-food industry.

ROLE OF BIOTECHNOLOGY IN FOOD INDUSTRY

Biotechnology in enzymes production: The industrial production of enzymes mainly involves the utilization of microorganisms. The microorganisms are cultured in enormous containers after which the desired enzymes are secreted into the medium in which the microorganism was fermented. The enzymes are secreted as a result of microbial activity in form of metabolites. It is with the help protein engineering techniques, which leads to the generation of unique enzymes.

The use of enzymes is done at industrial level processing of food items as well as enhancing its production. The food processing industries worldwide make use of the enzymes that are produced with the help of organisms that are genetically modified (*see* below). The enzymes thus produced comprises carbohydrases and proteases. In order to get greater production in a smaller amount of time, cloning of the genes involved in the enzyme production is done. These enzymes are used for various purposes such as production of cheese, making curd and adding flavors to the food items. In developed nations the major fraction of the enzymes used in food industry is proteases and carbohydrases, which makes more than 50% of the enzymes used.

Common genetically modified enzymes used in food industry

- Catalase used in mayonnaise production and it removes hydrogen peroxide.
- Chymosin useful in cheese production as it coagulates milk.
- Glucose oxidase is used in baking as it stabilizes the dough α-amylase converts starch into maltose and used in baking for sweetness Porotease used for meat tenderization process, baking and dairy products.

Biotechnology in enhancing taste: Biotechnology has permitted scientists to produce fruits and vegetables with better shelf life and taste. Genetically modified crops that have enhanced taste include the following: Seedless watermelon, cherries, tomato, eggplant and pepper, etc. In this the removal of seeds from the above food crops enhanced the soluble sugar content which in turn enhanced the sweetness.

Food and Nutrition Trends: 2020

Good carbs and bad carbs

Carbohydrates are regarded as the energy giving nutrient in our diet. But nowadays carbohydrates have been the targeted as a strategy to reduce overall calorie intake. Many of these diets focus on shifting intake of 'bad carbs', often referring to sugar or starches with minimal other nutritional value, to 'good carbs' like fruits, vegetables, whole grains, and legumes. Fiber is often a key differentiator between a 'good carb' and a 'bad carb'. This trend ties strongly with plant-based, such as the example of using vegetables as a base for pasta instead of refined starch.

Everyone love carb-based foods. Carb foods like bread or pasta are the major food which everyone likes and enjoys at every event of life. Innovations to deliver low-carb versions of these, that still taste good and deliver the nutrition consumers expect, is the important factors which are adopted by the food technologists. Whole grains and fiber still have a place across all product categories. They are health beneficial having good taste also.

Energy

Consumers prioritize the nutrition that affects them day-to-day, such as energy, stress, and sleep. When it comes to energy, the demand for energy has expanded beyond a morning cup of coffee or energy drinks. Energy means different things to different people. It can mean focus, mental stimulation, mood or even the ability to do physical labor or exercise. This means it is key to use the right solution for the category you are working on.

Plant-based

Natural foods are not only health beneficial but have good impact on our mood also. Now the trends have been shift to plant-based ice creams or yogurts, and plant-forward pastas. The major innovations in food industry are still largely based on nutrition and sustainability, and innovations in plant-based should be sure to deliver on these innovations. Food products with plant protein and vegetable-based pasta are just a couple of examples of this trend's power for good health.

Digestive wellness of foods

Good digestion is necessary for good health. Digestive wellness has been a high-priority trend for years, but it has been continually evolving. The key is to make sure a true digestive health benefit is being offered to consumers—foods that can help reduce feelings of gas, bloating, or more severe gastrointestinal symptoms are the focus in this

gluten-free to grain-free, and developing food products using low-carbohydrate, vegetable-based flours instead of grains in traditional foods.

Proteins

Consumers are now looking to replace these fat and carbohydrates with something healthy nutrient. Protein continues to serve this need due to its association with improving lean body mass, reducing hunger between meals, and the 'sportification' trend. People are looking for more protein in foods and beverages across categories, at increasing amounts. This trend ties strongly with plant-based. This can bring major taste challenges to foods and beverages, especially when using plant proteins, but strategies to improve taste of these proteins have continued to advance.

Nutritional Value

Nutritional value is one of the important factors which help in knowing that whether we are eating according to our requirement or helps in knowing the count of nutrient. Nutritional value written on any food item helps to select some alternative, which can satisfy taste with a balanced pattern. Therefore, the basic importance of nutrition value is to promote the selection of foods that can provide low calories, less saturated fats, and refined carbohydrate content in adequate amount.

Health benefits

Everyone knows good nutrition and physical activity can help maintain a healthy weight. But the benefits of good nutrition go beyond weight. Good nutrition can help in reducing the risk of some diseases, including heart disease, diabetes, stroke, some cancers, and osteoporosis. It is therefore necessary to know the health benefits of each item we purchase from the market or we prepare at home. Understanding the health benefits of food will help in managing the disease or will help in preventing the disease to occur.

Basic of Nutrition

Food is essential for survival of life and helps the body to function well and stay healthy. Mother Nature has given us a variety of healthy and nutritious foods. The food provided by our nature not only satisfies the hunger but also make life healthy as these food items are filled with the treasure of nutrients which make life healthy. The food is consumed for maintenance of health, growth and development. Food comprises various nutrients including protein, carbohydrate and fat that not only offer calories to fuel the body and give it energy but also play specific roles in maintaining health. Food also supplies micronutrients such as vitamins and minerals that do not provide calories but plays critical role in carrying out various body functions to keeps the body fit and healthy.

In every food the nutrients are present in varying proportions, which are needed for normal functioning of life processes. The food items are prepared by various processes and by combination of different food items which result in making the diet balanced.

▌ DEFINITION OF NUTRITION

Nutrition is defined as a science concerned with the role of food and nutrients in the maintenance of health.

According to Robinson (1982): Nutrition is *"the science of foods and nutrients, their action, interaction and balance in relationship to health and disease, the processes by which the organism ingests, digests, absorbs, transports and utilizes nutrients and disposes of their end product".*

According to WHO: Nutrition is the intake of food, considered in relation to the body's dietary needs.

Good nutrition: An adequate, well balanced diet combined with regular physical activity is a cornerstone of good health.

Poor nutrition: Poor nutrition can lead to reduced immunity, increased susceptibility to disease, impaired physical and mental development, and reduced productivity.

Nutrients: Nutrients are the essential components of food that are needed to be supplied to the body in adequate amounts. These include:

- Carbohydrates
- Proteins
- Fats
- Minerals
- Vitamins.

Nutritional Status: Nutritional status is the

status can be influenced by the intake of the nutrients.

RELATION BETWEEN HEALTH AND NUTRITION

Health is defined by the World Health Organization (WHO) as the *"State of complete physical, mental and social well-being and not merely the absence of disease or infirmity"*.

For leading a healthy life nutrition is very important. For achieving good health the nutritional status should be good and for achieving good nutritional status one need to take a healthy diet. The diet should contain all the nutrients in the correct proportion.

Essential requisites of good nutrition are:
- Optimal growth and development.
- Maintenance of the structural integrity and functional efficiency of body tissues.
- Good mental status.
- Ability to combat infections
- Healthy relations in environment
- Ability to cope up with difficult situations

ROLE OF NUTRITION IN LIFE

Nutrition is important for proper development of body. Due to lack of nutrition body becomes prone to get the diseases easily and nutritional disorders like night blindness, scurvy, anemia, bone disorders, etc. may also occur. Improper nutrition may weaken the body which results in feeling lethargic, mottled teeth, lack of energy, lack of interest in doing the activities, low immunity, dry hairs and skin. The improper diet lacking the important nutrients results in loss of internal and external power and the body function also retards. Good nutrition helps in providing the essential nutrients to the body such as proteins, carbohydrates, fats, minerals and vitamins which play important role in maintaining the structural integrity of the cells, but beside these nutrients there are some other nutrients which are also obtained from food and help in preventing the breakdown of tissues and also prevent free radical formation. These components are phytochemicals and antioxidants which have anti-inflammatory effects and prevent damage of cells from sun, pollution, smoke and from other, such as poor food intake. Good nutrition aids in digestion and absorption of food and the nutrients through the blood stream are adequately circulated in body and are utilized whenever needed. Good nutrition also affects our mental health. The ability of our mind to function well is the result of our nutritional intake. Good nutrition makes the mind fit and makes us able to take the decision and to solve out our day-to-day problems.

BALANCED DIET

A balanced diet needs to contain foods from all the main food groups in the correct proportions to provide the body with optimum nutrition.

According to Dr. JS Mclester: *Balanced diet is that which both in sickness and health will meet but not exceed a person's caloric needs and which is designed to provide as far as possible in liberal excess of body's calculated requirements of all nutritive essentials, notably proteins and vitamins.*

Balanced diet:
- *Provides 60–70% of calories from carbohydrates*
- *Provides 10–20% from proteins*
- *20–25% from fats*

Importance of Balanced Diet

Balanced diet is important because:
- It provides adequate energy which helps in doing daily activities of life and for carrying out the body mechanisms correctly.
- It helps in maintaining the normal growth and development of body, and also repairs the damaged tissues.

- It helps in regulation of all the body functions.
- The nutritional requirements of the body are adequately fulfilled.
- It helps in keeping the digestion proper and bowel movements occur well.
- All the chemical reactions of the body occur well.
- A balanced diet is necessary for keeping out the vitamin deficiencies which usually occur in the children of preschool period.
- For the nourishment of all the body organs.

CONCEPTS OF MALNUTRITION— UNDERNUTRITION AND OVER-NUTRITION

When a person does not eat a well balanced diet then the condition occur is malnutrition. Malnutrition occurs due to the deficiency of essential nutrients. Sometimes, it may occur due to the any long term illness or disease.

Malnutrition results in following:
- Stunting
- Reduced physical development
- Reduced mental development
- Risk of catching infections frequently.

According to World Health Organization (WHO): Malnutrition is a pathological state resulting from a relative or absolute deficiency or excess of one or more essential nutrients, this state being clinically manifested or detected only by biochemical, anthropometric or physiological tests.

Protein Energy Malnutrition (PEM)

When the diet lacks adequate amount of proteins and calories then the condition occur is malnutrition.

Following are the major forms of PEM:
  i. **Primary PEM:** Lack of adequate protein in the diet leads to primary PEM.

  ii. **Secondary PEM:** Secondary PEM is common problem in United States and is related to cancer, kidney failure, AIDS, inflammatory bowel disease, and illnesses reducing absorption and use of nutrients; depending on the patient's health, the organ may be negatively affected.

 iii. **Kwashiorkor:** This mainly occurs in the age group of 1–5 year of children. Lack of protein in diet leads to kwashiorkor. Kwashiorkor typically starts after the child has been weaned and breast milk has been replaced with a diet in low protein, although, it can occur in infants, if the mother is protein-deprived. Kwashiorkor can also occur due to parasites and infections that can interfere with nutritional status.

Causes of Kwashiorkor

Kwashiorkor is most common in areas where there is:
- Famine
- Low protein diets
- Limited food supply
- Milk allergies in infants
- Fad diets
- Low levels of education (when people do not understand how to eat a proper diet)

Symptoms of Kwashiorkor

- Changes in color of hair
- Increased infections due to low immunity
- Large belly
- Changes in pigment of skin
- Edema
- Fatigue
- Enlarged liver

Marasmus: Marasmus mainly occurs in children below age of 1 year. When the diet lacks both protein and energy in the diet, the condition occurs is marasmus. This lack of nutrition can range from a shortage of certain vitamins to complete starvation. Marasmus occurs most often in developing nations or in countries where poverty, along with inadequate food supplies and contaminated water, are prevalent. Marasmus often affects children in regions with high rates of poverty.

Causes of Marasmus

- Contaminated water supplies
- Chronic hunger
- Poor, unbalanced diet lacking in grains, fruits and vegetables, and protein
- Inadequate food supplies
- Other vitamin deficiencies (vitamin A, E or K)

Symptoms

The symptoms include:
- Chronic or persistent diarrhea
- Dizziness
- Unexplained weight loss
- Fatigue
- Change in level of consciousness or lethargy
- Full or partial paralysis of the legs
- Loss of bladder or bowel control
- Prolonged vomiting or diarrhea
- Retardation
- Wasting of muscles
- Swelling of legs and feet
- Wrinkled skin
- Abdomen protuberant
- Monkey face
- Increased appetite
- Infection is common.

Diet Therapy for Marasmus

A nutritious, well-balanced diet containing adequate calories, high protein, carbohydrates, minerals and vitamins should be given to the patient. The diet must includes food items such as fresh fruits and vegetables, grains and pulses.

Nutrition education of mothers is also a necessary part of treatment. The mothers should be told to continue breastfeeding for as long as possible as this helps in improving the nutritional status of the child.

Marasmic Kwashiorkor

The child shows a mixture of some of the features of marasmus and kwashiorkor. This is due to the varying nature of the dietary deficiency and the social factors responsible for the disease and presence or absence of infections.

Programmes for Preventing Malnutrition in India

Mid-day Meal Scheme

Mid-day Meal scheme was started on 15th August, 1995 with the goals to enhance enrolment, retention and attendance while simultaneously improving nutritional levels among children in school.

The main objectives of the scheme (as per the 2006 revision) are:
- To improve the nutritional status of children in classes one through five in government schools and government-aided schools.
- To encourage children from disadvantaged backgrounds to attend school regularly and to help them in concentrating in school activities.
- To provide nutritional support to students in drought-ridden areas throughout summer vacation.

Integrated Child Development Services

Integrated child development services (ICDS) comes under Ministry of Social Welfare and was started on 2nd October 1975, for childhood development. The main objective of the programme is to improve the health status of the children and to prevent the causes of child mortality, disability, morbidity and related malnutrition.

Objectives of ICDS

- To improve the nutritional status of pre-school children of 0–6 years of age group.
- To lay the foundation of proper psycho-logical development of the child.
- To reduce the incidence of mortality, morbidity malnutrition and school dropout.
- To achieve effective coordination of policy and implementation in various departments to promote child development.
- To enhance the capability of the mother to look after the normal health and nutritional needs of the child through proper nutrition and health education.

Special Nutrition Programme (SNP)

Another nutritional programme "SNP" was launched in the country in 1970–71. SNP provides supplementary feeding to the school children and to the expected and nursing mothers. Under this programme about 300 calories and 10 g of protein are provided to preschool children and about 500 calories and 25 g of protein to expect and nursing mothers for six days a week.

Balwadi Nutrition Programme

Balwadi refers to a place where, the children in the age group of 2½ to 5 years receive pre-primary education. The *balwadi* teachers are usually local women.

Balwadi also runs the nutrition programmes which come under the Department of Social Welfare which are meant for pre-school children. This programme was started in December 1970. The nutritional services are provided to the children in the age group of 3–5 years. Supplementary nutrition of 300 calories and 10 g of protein during 270 days for children attending *balwadis* are provided.

ROLE OF VITAMINS

In the field of health, the discovery of vitamins is a remarkable achievement. In 1906, English biochemist Sir Frederick Gowland Hopkins discovered that certain food factors which were important to health. The term vitamin was coined in 1912, by *Casimir Funk*. Funk originally coined the term "vitamine". Funk named the special nutritional parts of food as a "vitamine" after "vita" meaning life and "amine" from compounds found in the thiamine he isolated from rice husks. Vitamine was later shortened to vitamin. Together, Hopkins and Funk formulated the vitamin hypothesis of deficiency disease—that a lack of vitamins could make sick.

In 1905, the first scientist to determine that if special factors (vitamins) were removed from food disease occurred was Englishman, William Fletcher. Doctor Fletcher was researching the causes of the disease beriberi when he discovered that eating unpolished rice prevented beriberi and eating polished rice did not. William Fletcher believed that there were special nutrients contained in the husk of the rice.

Types of Vitamins

Water-soluble Vitamins

The important water-soluble vitamins are as follows:

Vitamin	Year of discovery	Function	Dietary sources	Deficiency
Vitamin A	Elmer V McCollum and M Davis discovered vitamin A during 1912–1914. In 1913,	Vitamin A is important for vision, healthy	Vitamin A from animal sources (retinol): Fortified milk, cheese,	Night blindness, perifollicular hyperkeratosis,

Contd.

Vitamin	Year of discovery	Function	Dietary sources	Deficiency
	Yale researchers, Thomas Osborne and Lafayette Mendel discovered that butter contained a fat-soluble nutrient soon known as vitamin A. Vitamin A was first synthesized in 1947.	skin and mucous membranes, bone and tooth growth, immune system health.	cream, butter, fortified margarine, eggs, liver. Beta-carotene (from plant sources): Leafy, dark green vegetables; dark orange fruits (apricots, cantaloupe) and vegetables (carrots, winter squash, sweet potatoes, pumpkin)	xerophthalmia, keratomalacia, increased morbidity and mortality in young children.
Vitamin D	In 1922, Edward Mellanby discovered vitamin D while researching a disease called rickets.	Important for proper absorption of calcium; stored in bones	Egg yolks, liver, fatty fish, fortified milk, fortified margarine. When exposed to sunlight, the skin can make vitamin D.	Rickets in children, osteoporosis in adults
Vitamin E	In 1922, University of California researchers, Herbert Evans and Katherine Bishop discovered vitamin E in green leafy vegetables.	Acts as anti-oxidant; protects cell walls	Polyunsaturated plant oils (soybean, corn, cottonseed, safflower); leafy green vegetables; wheat germ; whole-grain products; liver; egg yolks; nuts and seeds	RBC hemolysis, neurologic deficits
Vitamin K	Vitamin K was discovered by H Dam in 1929 in studying cholesterol metabolism in chicks. He noted a new deficiency syndrome in the young birds fed a fat deficient diet. The characteristic features were a lengthened blood clotting time, anemia and hemorrhage.	Important for proper blood clotting.	Green leafy vegetables and the cabbage family; milk; also produced in intestinal tract by bacteria.	Bleeding due to deficiency of prothrombin and other factors, osteopenia.

Fat-soluble Vitamins

Fat soluble vitamins are as follows:

Vitamin	Year of discovery	Function	Dietary sources	Deficiency
Vitamin B₁ (thiamine)	Casimir Funk discovered in 1912	Part of an enzyme needed for energy metabolism; important to nerve function	Pork, whole-grain or enriched breads and cereals, legumes, nuts and seeds	Beriberi (peripheral neuropathy, heart failure), Wernicke-Korsakoff syndrome

Contd.

Vitamin	Year of discovery	Function	Dietary sources	Deficiency
Vitamin B$_2$ (riboflavin)	DT Smith and EG Hendrick discovered B2 in 1926.	Part of an enzyme needed for energy metabolism; important for normal vision and skin health	Milk and milk products; leafy green vegetables; whole-grain, enriched breads and cereals	Cheilosis, angular stomatitis, corneal vascularization
Vitamin B$_3$ (niacin)	American, Conrad Elvehjem discovered in 1937.	Part of an enzyme needed for energy metabolism; important for nervous system, digestive system.	Meat, poultry, fish, whole-grain or enriched breads and cereals, vegetables (especially mushrooms, asparagus, and leafy green vegetables), peanut butter	Pellagra (dermatitis, glossitis, gastrointestinal and central nervous system dysfunction)
Vitamin B$_6$ (pyridoxine)	Paul Gyorgy discovered in 1934.	Part of an enzyme needed for protein metabolism; helps in formation of red blood cells (RBC)	Meat, fish, poultry, vegetables, fruits	Seizures, anemia, neuropathies, seborrheic dermatitis
Vitamin B$_{12}$ (cobalamin)	In the 1850s the English physician Thomas Addison described a lethal (pernicious) form of anaemia that could be related to pathological gastric mucosa and associated with the absence of acid in the stomach.	It helps in the production of DNA and RNA. Vitamin B$_{12}$ also works closely with vitamin B$_9$, also called folate or folic acid, to help make red blood cells and to help iron work better in the body	Meat, poultry, fish, seafood, eggs, milk and milk products; not found in plant foods	Megaloblastic anemia, neurologic deficits (confusion, paresthesias, ataxia)
Vitamin C (ascorbic acid)	In 1747, Scottish naval surgeon James Lind discovered that an nutrient (now known to be vitamin C) in citrus foods prevented scurvy. It was rediscovered by Norwegians, A Hoist and T Froelich in 1912. Vitamin C was the first vitamin to be artificially synthesized in 1935.	It acts an antioxidant, part of an enzyme needed for protein metabolism; important for immune system health; aids in iron absorption	Found only in fruits and vegetables, especially citrus fruits, vegetables in the cabbage family, cantaloupe, strawberries, peppers, tomatoes, potatoes, lettuce, papayas, mangoes, kiwifruit.	Scurvy (hemorrhages, loose teeth, gingivitis, bone defects)

Contd.

Vitamin	Year of discovery	Function	Dietary sources	Deficiency
	A process invented by Dr Tadeusz Reichstein, of the Swiss Institute of Technology in Zurich.			

▌ROLE OF MINERALS

Minerals are inorganic substances that are found in various foods. They are essential nutrients that the body needs to survive and carry out daily functions and processes. Our body receives minerals by eating different foods. Minerals keep us healthy and have key roles in several body functions. We require these important nutrients from our daily diet.

The minerals in our diet are essential for a variety of important functions in our body. They are important for building strong bones and teeth, blood, skin, hair, nerve function, muscle and for metabolic processes such as those that turn the food we eat into energy. This means that minerals are needed for the body to work properly, for growth and development, and overall, for **maintaining normal health.**

The important minerals that are essential to human health are: Calcium, phosphorus, magnesium, sodium, potassium, chloride, sulfur, iron, manganese, copper, iodine, zinc, fluoride and selenium. These 14 essential minerals are essential for the growth and production of bones, teeth, hair, blood, nerves, skin, vitamins, enzymes and hormones and the healthy functioning of nerve transmission, blood circulation, fluid regulation, cellular integrity, energy production and muscle contraction.

Different minerals are required in different amounts but they are all essential. Minerals are grouped depending on how much they are needed on a daily basis.

On this basis minerals are of two types:

Macro-minerals: Minerals that are needed in larger amounts on a daily basis are known as the minerals, macro-minerals or major minerals.

Micro-minerals: Minerals that are needed in smaller amounts are known as micro-minerals or "trace elements".

Children, pregnant and breastfeeding mothers and older people may need to adjust their intake depending on the type of mineral. It is also important to note that excessively high intakes of minerals can be toxic (harmful).

▌ Important Functions of Minerals

▌ Bone and Teeth Health

Our skeleton provides motility, protection and support for the body. It also stores minerals and other nutrients. Though they appear hard and unyielding, our bones are actually constantly being reabsorbed and reformed by our body. Several minerals make up the hard architecture of our bones. Calcium is the most abundant mineral in our body and is found in bones and blood. Along with the minerals phosphorus and magnesium, calcium gives our bones strength and density.

This mineral also builds and maintains strong, healthy teeth. Calcium deficiency due to poor nutrition or illness can lead to osteoporosis, a condition in which the bones become brittle and less dense, increasing the risk of fractures.

Foods that are rich in calcium include milk and other dairy products, green, leafy vegetables and canned fish with bones.

▌ Energy Production

Oxygen is required to produce energy that is necessary for every bodily function and process. Red blood cells or erythrocytes carry oxygen to each of our infinite cells, where it is used to generate energy. Red blood cells contain a heme or iron component that binds to oxygen so that it can be transported.

Without iron which is mineral, oxygen could not be attached to the blood cells without iron and the body would not be able to produce the energy necessary for life.

Iron is an essential mineral, and failing to get enough from diet can lead to a condition called anemia, which causes weakness and fatigue. This mineral is primarily found in the blood, and it is also stored in our liver, spleen, bone marrow and muscles.

Nerve and Muscle Function

Potassium is another important mineral which is found in tomatoes, green leafy vegetables, citrus fruits, bananas, dates, and legumes such as peas and lentils. Potassium nutrient is important to keep muscles and the nervous system functioning normally. Potassium helps to maintain the correct water balance in the cells of our nerves and muscles. Without this essential mineral, the nerves could not generate an impulse to signal body to move, and the muscles of our heart, organs and body would not be able to contract and relax.

Immune Health

Zinc is a trace mineral that is required in small quantities. Zinc is important for keeping our immune system strong and helps our body fight infections, heal wounds and repair cells. Another mineral called selenium is also needed in small amounts for immune health. A deficiency of selenium has been linked to an increased risk of heart disease and even some types of cancers.

Macro-minerals, their functions and food sources

Mineral	Function	Common food sources	Deficiency diseases
Calcium	Plays important role in formation of bones and teeth and helps keep them strong. Calcium also helps the muscles of our heart to work properly.	Milk, cheese, yogurt, calcium fortified non-dairy beverages, tofu with added calcium	Arthritis, high blood pressure and osteoporosis. Rickets in children.
Phosphorus	It plays an important role in the growth, maintenance, and repair of cells. It maintains the pH level (acidity-alkalinity) of the blood. It helps in reducing the pain of arthritis. It is essential for speedy recovery of burn victims. Helps in cancer prevention.	Milk, yogurt, cottage cheese, pork, hamburger, tuna, lobster, chicken, sunflower seeds, peanuts, pine nuts, peanut butter, bran flakes, whole wheat bread, noodles, rice, white bread, potatoes, corn, peas, french fries, broccoli, milk chocolate and soda beverages (due to the phosphoric acid added as a preservative).	Rickets, osteoporosis, stiff joints and pain in the bones. The deficiency can also cause anxiety, irritability, sensitive skin, stress, tiredness and weak teeth, etc.

Contd.

Macro-minerals, their functions and food sources (*Contd.*)

Mineral	Function	Common food sources	Deficiency diseases
	It is essential for building of strong bones and skeletal structure. It maintains heart regularity.		
Magnesium	Keeps nerves and muscles strong Helps form bones and teeth.	Spinach and Bran cereals and wheat germ Dried beans, peas and lentils such as chickpeas, nuts and seeds such as almonds, cashews, pumpkin, sunflower and flax seeds.	Heart disease, diabetes and osteoporosis.
Potassium	Potassium is needed for growth, building muscles, transmission of nerve impulses, heart activity, etc. It assists in muscle contractions and in maintaining appropriate levels of fluid and the electrolyte balance in the body cells. Potassium also plays an important role in the conduction of nerve impulses and enables the body to convert glucose into energy, which is then stored in reserve by the muscles and liver. Potassium is essential for maintaining fluid balance in the body.	Bananas, broccoli, tomatoes, potatoes with skins, kiwi, leafy green vegetables, broccoli citrus fruits, oranges, dried fruits, dates, apricots, avocado, beans, peas, lentils, and peanuts are rich sources of potassium.	Weakness Scarring of heart muscle, irregular heart-beat or heart failure Hypertrophy of kidneys Paralysis of muscle Retarded bone growth.
Sodium	Sodium is important for the manufacture of hydrochloric acid in the stomach, which protects the body from any infections that may be present in food. It is required for maintaining blood pressure. The important function of sodium is to regulate fluids and acid–base balance in the body.	Sodium is found in table salt, ajinomoto, sauces, etc.	Fatigue, cramping legs, muscle weakness, slow reflexes, acne, dry skin, mood changes and irregular heartbeat.

Macro-minerals, their functions and food sources (*Contd.*)

Mineral	Function	Common food sources	Deficiency diseases
	Sodium is required for nerve transmission and muscle contraction. Sodium is important for treatment of diarrhea, leg cramps, dehydration and fever.		

Micro-minerals, their functions and food sources

Mineral	Function	Common food sources	Deficiency diseases
Iron	Carries oxygen to all parts of our body Prevents us from feeling tired.	Meat, fish, poultry, firm tofu, dried beans, peas, like soybeans, chickpeas, split pea, lentils, nuts and seeds, organ meats such as liver. Iron fortified grain products like flour, bread, pasta and breakfast cereal.	Anemia
Zinc	Maintains a healthy immune system Helps in rapid wound healing Helps the body in utilizing other nutrients. Needed for growth and development.	Yogurt, milk, cheese Dried beans like kidney, navy, pinto and soybeans, lentils, pumpkin seeds and sunflower seeds, liver, meat, poultry, fish and seafood.	Allergies Night blindness Loss of smell Falling hair White spots under fingernails Skin problems Sleep disturbances
Copper	Copper is important for the formation of collagen. Copper is important component of cyto-chromeoxidase, controls intracellular energy production.	Good sources include cocoa, liver, kidney, peas and raisins. Molluscs and shellfish are rich sources of copper, as are betel leaves and other nuts.	The deficiency of copper leads to Menkes' syndrome, Wilson's disease, Kwashiorkor and neutropenia.

Contd.

Micro-minerals, their functions and food sources (*Contd.*)

Mineral	Function	Common food sources	Deficiency diseases
	It helps in controlling various hormone levels in the body. Prevents free radical formation. Copper is important for fatty acid metabolism. It helps in maintaining the normal hemoglobin level in the body.		
Iodine	Iodine is important micro-nutrient which is required for normal growth and development of human brain and body. It is important for the synthesis of triiodothyronine (T3) and thyroxine (T4). The thyroid hormones play an important role in the growth and development.	Iodine is added to most table salt so people generally get the required amount from just one tea-spoon of iodized salt. Other iodine sources include eggs, milk, sea fish and sea food, sea vege-table—such as kelp, seaweed, asparagus, etc. Fruits and vegetables grown in coastal regions, are other good sources of iodine.	Acne, bad circu-lation, confused thinking, cretinism fatigue, goiter, hor-monal imbalance, menstrual diffi-culties miscarriages, scaly or dry skin, sterility, weight gain and weight loss, etc.
Selenium	Selenium is required in the diet for the proper func-tioning of immune system and for preventing free radical formations. It also protects against heart weakness and degene-ration and is essential for the production of thyroid hormones. Selenium is found to have cancer reducing effect.	Red meat, chicken, turkey, liver, fish, shellfish, dark green leafy vegetables, whole grains, eggs, onions, brazil nuts, walnuts, brewer's yeast, wheat germ, pasta, noodles, rice, cottage cheese, cheddar cheese and garlic are all good sele-nium sources.	Malabsorption, but that too is rare.
Fluoride	Fluorine is important for preventing the teeth from decaying. It is also invol-ved in imparting stability to bone and enamel tissue.	The chief source of fluorine is drinking water which should contain 1 part per million (ppm) of fluorine.	Cavities and weakened tooth enamel

Contd.

Micro-minerals, their functions and food sources (*Contd.*)

Mineral	Function	Common food sources	Deficiency diseases
	Thus, it prevents dental caries and osteoporosis.	Sea fish is also a good source of fluorine.	
Chromium	Chromium is needed for energy, maintains stable blood sugar levels.	Some of the best dietary sources of chromium include egg yolks, bread made from whole wheat, fruit juices, hard cheeses, lean beef, brewer's yeast, molasses and liver.	Anxiety, fatigue, glucose intolerance, inadequate metabolism of amino acids, and an increased risk of arteriosclerosis.

Food Additives

Food additives are the substances which are added in food during its preparation. Food additives are added for preserving flavor or for enhancing taste and appearance.

Food additives when added in foods they add enjoyment and act as appetizing, nutritious, fresh, and palatable foods. Although additives are added in small quantities in food but their impact is great.

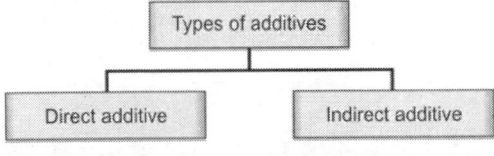

Direct additive: This category belongs to those food additives which are added in food for a specific purpose. For example, xanthan gum—used in chocolate milk, bakery fillings, puddings and other foods to add texture—is a direct additive.

Indirect additive: The indirect food additives which are added in food in trace amounts due to its packaging, storage or other handling.

▌FUNCTIONS OF FOOD ADDITIVES

Additives perform various functions in foods. Additives are beneficial for the food producer as well as for the consumer. Additives improve the appearance of food product and improve the quality and nutritive values of food and thus make the food acceptable.

Important functions played by food additives are as follows:

- For safety and freshness.
- Maintaining or improving nutritional quality.
- To maintain or improve product safety or quality.
- Aids in processing or preparations.
- Enhancing sensory characteristics of the food.
- Improving the texture of food and thus makes food acceptable.
- Additives may help in enriching the food or replacing nutrients that may have been lost during processing.
- They are also used as preservative agent.

▌MAJOR FOOD ADDITIVES

1. Preservatives or antimicrobial substances
2. Acids
3. Sweeteners
4. Emulsifiers
5. Anticaking agents
6. Antifoaming
7. Colors

8. Stabilizers
9. Antioxidants
10. Flour improvers
11. Flavors enhancers
12. Leavening agents
13. Nutritive additives
14. Tracer gas
15. Thickeners

Categories

Food additives can be divided into several groups with different functions. The functions and examples are as follows:

S. No.	Food additive	Function	Example
1.	Preservative or antimicrobial substances	Prevent food from spoiling due to mold, bacteria and other microorganisms	Salt, sugar, vinegar (natural), benzoic acid, esters of p-hydroxy acid or salicylic acid sulphites, sodium benzoate and sorbic acid
2.	Acids	They make taste sharper	Vinegar, citric acid, tartaric acid
3.	Sweeteners	They are non-nutritive and provide less than 2% caloric value of sucrose per equivalent unit of sweetening capacity when used to sweeten foods	Aspartame, Acesulfame-K
4.	Emulsifiers	These allow the water and oil to be remaining in mixed form	Lecithin, sodium phosphates, poly-oxyethylenes
5.	Anticaking agents	Prevent lumping and caking by absorbing moisture	Carbonates and phosphates of Ca and Mg, silicates of Ca, Mg, Al and Na, SiO_2, palmitic and stearic acid.
6.	Colors	Provide, retain and increase the color of food	Annatto, carotene, fast green, chlorophyll
7.	Stabilizers/jelling agents	Helps in giving firm texture to food	Pectin and agar
8.	Antioxidants	Prevents rancidity of foods caused by exposure to oxygen	Lecithin, vitamin C, citric acid, tartaric acid, gallic acid
9.	Flour improvers	For toughening of dough and for maintaining texture	Chlorine gas, benzoyl peroxide
10.	Flavor enhancers	For enhancing the aroma of food	Monosodium glutamate
11.	Leavening agents	For increasing the volume of dough or batter, gives dough fluffy structure. Also helps in production of carbon di-oxide gas in baked goods	Baking powder and sodium bicarbonate

Contd.

Contd.

S. No.	Food additive	Function	Example
12.	Nutritive additives	These help in preventing nutrients loss occur during processing of food	Iron, calcium, vitamin A, vitamin D, iodine
13.	Tracer gas	Tracer gas is allowed for package integrity testing to prevent foods from being exposed to atmosphere, for increasing shelf life	Carbon dioxide
14.	Thickeners	Thickeners are added to the mixture, increase viscosity without substantially modifying its other properties	Arrowroot, cornstarch, sodium pyropshosphate

Cooking of Food

Food is very important for the survival of life. Nature has given us various nutritious food items. Some foods are eaten as such that is in raw form but some foods cannot be eaten raw and requires some extra preparation so that taste and nutritional quality is enhanced.

Food preparation is an important step in meeting the nutritional needs of the family. Food preparation is done for enhancing the food appearance and taste. Fruits, vegetables and nuts can be eaten raw but there are various foods which require cooking. The process of subjecting food to the action of heat is termed as cooking.

OBJECTIVES OF COOKING FOOD

- *Removal of microorganisms:* Heating food above 40°C, the growth of bacteria decreases rapidly.
- *Improving digestibility:* During cooking all the connective tissues of meat and the coarse fiber of cereals, pulses and vegetables softens so that the digestive period is shortened and the gastrointestinal tract is less subjected to irritation.
- *Food quality is improved:* The color, appearance, flavor, texture and taste of food are enhanced when the food is cooked.
- *Variety in food is added:* One food can be prepared in several ways. For example,

wheat can be made into chapatis, puri, paratha or halwa.

- *Food consumption is increased:* During cooking improvement in texture and flavor is increased, therefore consumption of food is also increased.
- *Increase in nutritional quality:* Cooking of food results in improvement of nutritional quality of food. For example, cooking increases the quality protein by making some amino acids available to the body.

METHODS OF COOKING FOOD

During cooking of food heat is transferred by conduction, convection, radiation or microwave energy. Cooking occurs by moist and dry heat.

Cooking food by moist heat: Cooking of food by this method involves water and steam.

Cooking of food by dry heat: Cooking of food by this method involves air or fat.

Cooking by moist heat: This method of cooking involves:

- Boiling
- Pressure cooking
- Stewing
- Steaming
- Poaching
- Blanching

Cooking by dry heat: This method of cooking involves:

- Roasting
- Grilling
- Toasting
- Baking
- Sauteing
- Frying

Cooking by applying both—moist and dry heat:

Braising

Cooking Food by Moist Heat

Boiling

In boiling food is immersed in water at 100°C and the water is maintained at that temperature till the food become tender. Rice, egg, pulses, meat, roots and tubers are cooked by boiling.

Advantages

- Boiling is simple method of cooking and no special skills and equipment are required.
- By this method uniform cooking can be achieved.

Disadvantages

- Damage to the structure and texture of food may occur due to continuous boiling.
- Loss of heat labile nutrients such as B and C vitamins if the water is discarded.
- Boiling is time-consuming and loss of fuel occurs.
- Loss of water soluble pigments may result in loss of color of food.

Pressure Cooking

Cooking food in steam under pressure is known as pressure cooking. The equipment used for this cooking is pressure cooker. The steam can be raised above 100°C and cooking time is reduced. Food such as pulses, rice, roots and tubers, meat are pressure cooked.

Advantages

- Pressure cooking requires less time to cook so that its time saving process.
- Less loss of nutrient and flavor.
- Different items can be cooked in same time so fuel and time are saved.
- Less chance for burning and scorching.
- Constant attention is not required.

Disadvantages

- Knowledge of the usage, care and maintenance of cooker is required to prevent accidents.
- Requires careful watch during cooking to prevent over cooking.

Stewing

Stewing is a slow method of cooking. In this process the food is simmered in a pan using small quantities of water so that only half the food is covered in water. The liquid is brought to boiling point and the heat is reduced to maintain simmering temperatures (82°–90°C). The food above the liquid is cooked by the steam generated within the pan. The foods such as apple, meat, vegetables like roots and tubers and legumes are stewed.

Advantages

- Loss of nutrients does not occur.
- Flavor of food is retained.

Disadvantage

Time-consuming process.

Steaming

Foods are cooked in steam. Steam is generated from vigorously boiling water or liquid in a pan so that the food is completely surrounded by steam and not in contact with the water or liquid. The water should be boiled before the food is placed in the steamer. The food gets cooked at 100°C. Steaming is done in special equipment designated for the purpose, e.g. idli cooker.

Advantages

- Not requires constant attention.
- Less loss of nutrients.
- Foods cooked by steaming are easily digestible.
- Less chance of scorching of food.
- Foods are fluffy and have good texture.
- Foods have good flavor.

Disadvantages

- Special equipment is required.
- Whole grains are not prepared by this method.

Poaching

Cooking food in minimum amount of water at a temperature of 80°–85°C is poaching. Foods such as eggs, fish and fruits are cooked by poaching. Eggs are poached by adding a little salt or vinegar to the liquid and temperature of coagulation is lowered. Eggs get cooked quickly by poaching.

Advantages

- Very quick method of cooking.
- Easily digestible since no fat is used.

Disadvantages

- It is bland in taste.
- Water-soluble nutrients may be leached into the water.

Blanching

The foods which have outer coverings are peeled off without making them tender by the process called blanching. In this process the food items are dipped in boiling water for 1–2 minutes depending on the texture of the food. During this process the skin or the outer covering of foods are peeled easily without making the food soft. In blanching the food are immersed in boiling water for some time. This results in loosening of the outer skin or can be peeled off easily.

Advantages

- The enzymes are destroyed easily that cause spoilage.
- Digestibility is improved.
- Texture, color and flavor of food are improved.

Disadvantage

Blanching results in loss of nutrients.

COOKING FOOD BY DRY HEAT

Roasting

Cooking food without covering it is called roasting. Food is roasted in a baked metal, in sand or in hot ashes in an oven. Foods such as chapati, nan, breads, corn flakes, groundnuts, cashewnuts, walnuts, etc. are roasted.

Advantages

- Roasting is quick method of cooking.
- The appearance, flavor and texture of the food is improved.
- Spices are easily powdered if they are first roasted.

Disadvantages

- Food can be scorched due to carelessness.
- Attention is required.

Grilling

Grilling or broiling refers to the cooking of food by exposing it to direct heat. In this method food is placed above or in between a red hot surface. Papads, corn, phulkas, chicken can be prepared by this method.

Advantages

- Enhances flavor, appearance and taste of the product.
- It requires less time to cook.
- Minimum fat is used.

Disadvantage

Constant attention is required to prevent charring.

Baking

In baking, the food gets cooked in an oven or oven-like appliance by dry heat. The temperature range maintained in an oven is 120°–260°C. The food is usually kept uncovered in a container greased with a fat coated paper. Bread, cake, biscuits, pastries and meat are prepared by this method.

Advantages

- Unique flavor in food is developed.
- Foods become light and fluffy.
- Uniform and bulk cooking can be achieved. For example, bun, bread.
- Texture is improved.

Disadvantages

- Oven is required.
- Baking requires special skills for achieving ideal texture, flavor and color characteristics.
- Baking requires careful monitoring for prevention of scorching.

Toasting

Toasting is a process by which bread slices are kept under the grill or between the two heated elements to brown from both sides of the bread at the same time. This can be adjusted to give the required degree of brownness through temperature control.

Advantages

- Toasting is easy and quick method of cooking.
- Flavor is improved.

Disadvantages

- Special equipment is required for toasting.
- For prevention of charring careful monitoring is needed.

Sauteing

The food is lightly tossed in a little oil just enough to cover the base of the pan. The pan is covered with a lid and the flame or intensity of heat is reduced. The food is allowed to cook till it becomes tender in its own steam. The food is tossed occasionally, or turned with a spatula to enable all the pieces to come in contact with the oil and get cooked evenly. The product obtained by this method is slightly moist and tender but without any liquid or gravy. Foods generally tossed are vegetables which are used as side dishes in a menu these are cooked by sauteing. Sauteing can be combined with other methods to produce variety in meals.

Advantages

- This method requires less time.
- This is a simple technique of cooking.
- Minimum oil is used.

Disadvantage

Constant attention is needed as there is chance of scorching or burning.

Frying

In this method, the food items are cooked by bringing them into contact with larger amount of hot fat. The food items are totally immersed in hot oil, this process is called deep fat frying. Food items such as pakoda, samosa, chips, are examples of deep fat fried foods. In shallow fat frying, only a little fat is used and the food is turned in order that both sides are browned. For example, parathas, puris, etc.

Advantages

- Very quick method of cooking.
- The calorific values of food are increased.
- Taste and texture of foods are improved.
- Gives attractive appearance to foods.

Disadvantages

- Careful monitoring is required as food easily gets charred when the smoking temperature is not properly maintained.
- The food may become soggy due to too much oil absorption.
- Sometimes the same oil is repeated for heating which have ill effects on health.

Cooking by Applying Both—Moist and Dry Heat

Braising

Combination of method of roasting and stewing in a pan with a tight-fitting lid is braising. Flavorings and seasonings are added in the food and food is allowed to cook gently.

Food preparations prepared by combination methods are:

Cutlet—boiling and deep frying.
Upma—roasting and boiling.

MICROWAVE COOKING

Microwave cooking is the advanced form of cooking, which is done by electromagnetic waves of radiant energy with wavelengths in the range of 250×10^6 to 7.5×10^9 Angstroms. In microwave, the electronic device generator called magnetron generates radiant energy of high frequency. A simple microwave oven consists of a metal cabinet into which the magnetron is inserted. The cabinet is equipped with a metal fan that distributes the microwave throughout the cabinet. Food placed in the oven is heated from all directions. In microwave ovens moist and liquid foods can be rapidly heated. Food items should be kept in containers made of plastic, glass or chinaware which does not contain metallic substances. These containers help in transmitting the microwaves and do not absorb or reflect them.

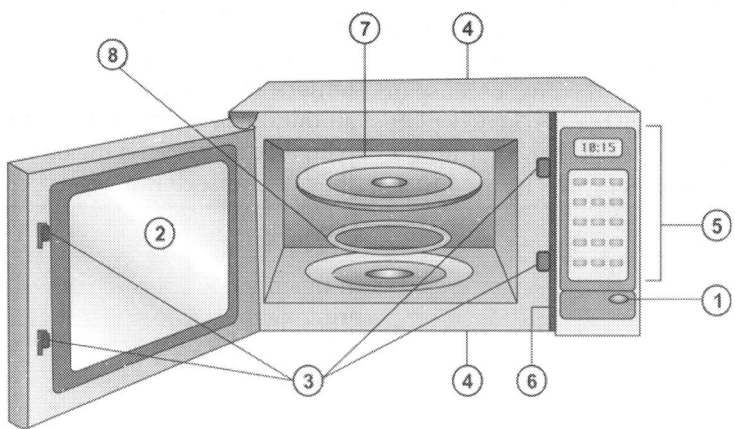

1. Door release button; 2. See through oven window; 3. Door safety lock system; 4. External air vents; 5. Control panel; 6. Identification plate; 7. Glass tray; and 8. Roller ring

Source: Srilakshmi B (2003). Food Science, New Age International (P) Publishers Limited, Chennai.

Advantages

- Quick method and saves time.
- Easiest method of cooking food.
- Uniform cooking is achieved.
- Flavors of food are enhanced.

Disadvantages

- Due to short period of cooking, food does not become brown unless the microwave has a browning unit.
- Chapati, tandoori roti cannot be cooked.
- Deep frying cannot be done in it.
- Careful operation is required.

SOLAR COOKING

Solar cooker works on solar energy. Solar cooker can directly utilize solar energy or can use deflected solar energy from a large concentration rays surface. Solar cooker consists of a well-insulated box, the inside of which is painted dull black and is covered by one or more transparent covers. The purpose of these transparent covers is to trap heat inside the solar cooker. These covers allow the radiation from the sun to come inside but do not allow the heat from the hot black absorbing plate to come out of the box. Because of this, the temperature of the blackened plate inside the box increases and can heat up the space inside the temperature up to 140°C

which is adequate for cooking. The second type of solar cooker uses a lens or a reflector suitably designed to concentrate the solar radiation over a small area. This cooker is able to provide higher temperatures on its absorbing surface when suitably designed but is usually more expensive than the box cooker.

The outer box: The outer box of a solar cooker may be made of wood, iron sheet or fibre reinforced plastic having suitable dimensions.

The inner box: The inner box can be made from galvanized iron or mild steel or aluminium sheet. All the four sides and the bottom of the inner box which are exposed to the sun are coated with black paint.

Mirror: Mirror is used in a solar cooker to increase the radiation input on the absorbing surface. Sunlight which falls on the mirror gets reflected from it and enters the box after passing through the glass covers. This radiation is in addition to the radiation entering the box directly and helps to quicken the cooking process by raising the inside temperature of the cooker. The use of a mirror can enhance the solar radiation input to the cooker by about 50%.

Cooking containers: The cooking containers with covers are generally made of aluminum or stainless steel. The containers are painted dull black on the outer surface so that they also absorb radiation directly.

Preserving the Food

FOOD PRESERVATION

The science that deals with the process of prevention of decay or spoilage of food thus allowing it to be stored in a fit condition for future use is food preservation.

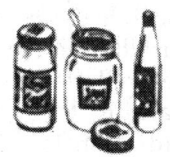

Food preservation is important task as it helps in saving the food from spoilage and makes it fit for consumption at the time of scarcity or for future needs.

SPOILAGE OF FOOD

Food spoilage is a state in which the food or its quality is deteriorated. Food is deprived of its good or effective qualities. Spoilage of food starts from the time it is harvested, slaughtered or manufactured and cause undesirable changes in the physical and chemical characteristics of food.

Causes of Food Spoilage

- Growth of microorganisms.
- Chemical reactions in food.
- Inappropriate temperatures for a given food.
- Moisture gain or loss.
- Reaction with oxygen and light.

- Insects and rodents.
- Enzymatic reactions in food.

Importance of Food Preservation

Food preservation is important for:
1. For keeping the food available throughout the year.
2. For increasing the distribution of food.
3. For transporting it from one place to another.
4. For saving money; if the food will be available in adequate amount then the price of food will be lowered and everyone will be able to purchase it.
5. For adding variety in food.
6. Keeping food for longer period of time.

PRINCIPLES OF FOOD PRESERVATION

1. Prevention or delay of microbial decomposition.
   a. By keeping out microorganisms (asepsis)
   b. By removal of microorganisms (e.g. filtration)
   c. By hindering the growth and activity of microorganisms, e.g. refrigeration, dehydration, addition of chemical preservatives.

d. By killing microorganisms, e.g. boiling, irradiation.

2. Prevention or delay of self-decomposition of food.

   a. By destruction or inactivation of enzymes, e.g. by blanching. The steaming or boiling of fruits or vegetables in water for a few minutes to inactivate natural enzymes and facilitates removal of skin is known as blanching.

   b. By prevention or delay of purely chemical reactions, e.g. prevention of oxidation by the use of antioxidants.

3. Prevention of damage caused by insects, animals and mechanical causes.

METHODS OF FOOD PRESERVATION

There are various methods employed for keeping the food preserved. They are as follows.

Home-based Methods of Preserving Foods

Foods can be preserved at home by the following methods:

   a. Dehydration
   b. Lowering temperature
   c. Increasing temperature
   d. Using preservatives

Dehydration

The word dehydration means removal of water or moisture from foods. The home method of dehydration is sun drying. Foods such as papads, green leafy vegetables (methi, pudina, corriander, etc.) cauliflower, grapes, amla, onion, raw mango, etc. are sun-dried. Some foods needed cooking before drying. For example, potato chips, papad, banana, chips, wadis, etc. are cooked before drying. The most appropriate weather to dry foods is when the air is dry and there is strong sunshine.

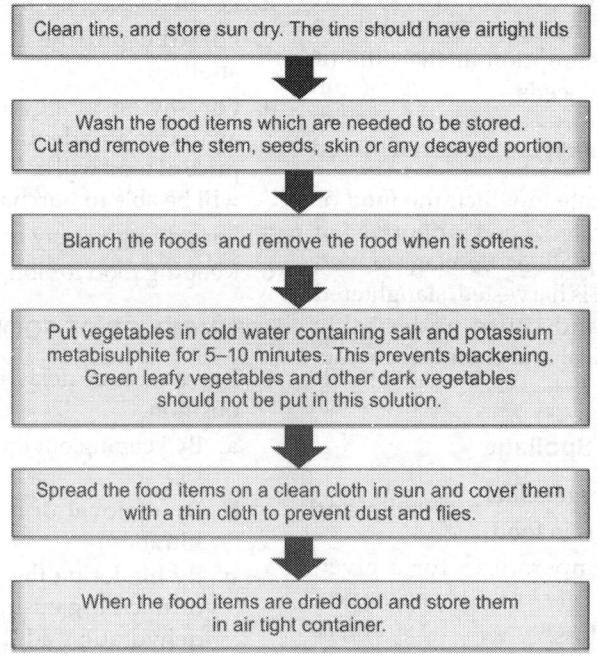

Clean tins, and store sun dry. The tins should have airtight lids

Wash the food items which are needed to be stored. Cut and remove the stem, seeds, skin or any decayed portion.

Blanch the foods and remove the food when it softens.

Put vegetables in cold water containing salt and potassium metabisulphite for 5–10 minutes. This prevents blackening. Green leafy vegetables and other dark vegetables should not be put in this solution.

Spread the food items on a clean cloth in sun and cover them with a thin cloth to prevent dust and flies.

When the food items are dried cool and store them in air tight container.

Steps in dehydration

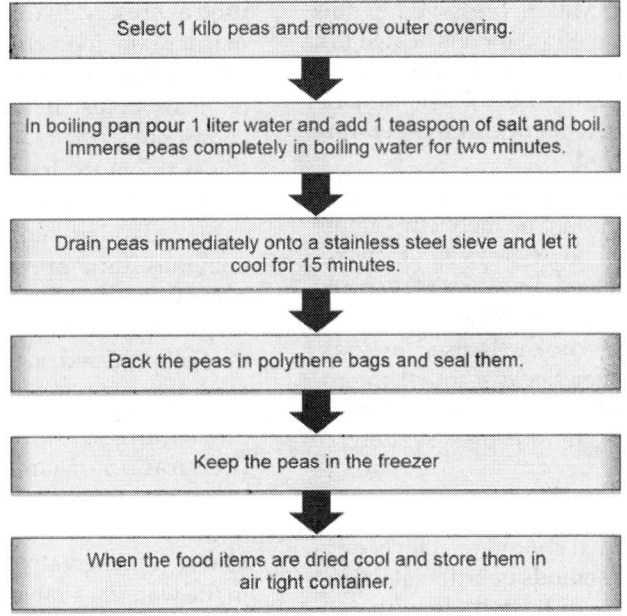

Freezing of peas

Lowering Temperature

Application of low temperature results in slowing down the microbial and enzymatic action. The food is thus prevented from spoilage. At home, this method is applied with the help of refrigerator. Foods can be preserved at low temperature by:

1. Refrigeration $-4°$ to $7°C$
2. Cold storage $-1°$ to $-4°C$
3. Freezing $-18°C$ or below

Preservation by this method varies with the type of food and temperature. The lower the temperature, longer is the duration for which food can be preserved.

Precautions While Freezing Fruits and Vegetables

1. Polythene bags used for preserving the peas and other food items should be strong so that they can withstand expansion of foods on freezing.

2. The food once brought out of the freezer and up to room temperature should not be refrozen.
3. Small packets should be prepared; as food once thawed (process by which something frozen is brought to room temperature without applying artificial heat must be consumed). So there is less chance of the unrequired food material being spoilt. This also helps to avoid refreezing of the unutilized food material.
4. Exclude the air carefully and completely from the package before sealing.
5. The freezer should not be opened too frequently.

Increasing Temperature

The microorganisms and enzymes are destroyed by increasing the temperature so that the food is not spoiled.

There are mainly two methods of preserving foods by using high temperature:
1. Pasteurization
2. Sterilization

1. *Pasteurization:* Milk is preserved by this method. In this method food is heated to a high temperature and then quickly cooled. The microorganisms are not able to withstand the sudden change in temperature and are destroyed.

2. *Sterilization:* Sterilization means free from any living organism. The high temperature used in this method destroys all the microorganisms in the food. The foods are exposed to high temperature for longer time.

When a pressure cooker is used to cook, the food lasts longer because most microorganisms get destroyed. Bottles and other equipment are sterilized for preservation.

Drying by Mechanical Driers

This process is used at commercial level or in an industry. Most methods of artificial drying involve the passage of heated air with controlled relative humidity over the food to be dried or the passage of the food through such air. Fruits, vegetables, nuts, fish and meat can be successfully preserved by this method. In the dehydration process, artificial drying methods (e.g. spray drier) are used for drying foods. Although it is expensive when compared to natural sun-drying procedures, it is very advantageous because the temperature and relative humidity can be manipulated.

Spray Drying

Milk and egg are dried to a powder in spray driers in which the liquid is atomized and sprayed into a hot air stream for almost instant drying.

Preservation by using Preservatives

Preservatives: The substances that are added to foods to make it last for a longer time is called a preservative. There are two types of preservatives:

1. Natural Preservatives

- *Salt:* Salt is used for adding taste at home during preparation of pickle. But it is also used as preservative. Increasing the quantity of salt in the food changes its composition. Due to the presence of salt in the food, osmosis takes place. As a result, water comes out of the food. When there is no or less water in the food, the microorganisms are not able to grow and the food becomes safe. Salt also reduces the activity of enzymes, thus preventing the food from getting spoilt. Salt is used as a preservative in pickles, chutney, sauce, canned food, etc. Salt is rubbed on fish which helps to preserve it.

- *Sugar:* Sugar is often used during the preparation of jams, jellies, murabbas, squashes, pickle, chutney, etc., sugar is added to these foods not only for taste but also as a preservative. The sugar dissolves in the water available in the food item. This results in less water being available for the growth of microorganisms. Hence, the food becomes safe.

- *Acids:* Lemon juice, vinegar, citric acid, etc. are the natural acids which are used for the preparation of pickle and other food items. Vinegar is used to preserve onions, tomato ketchup; lemon juice is used in pickles; citric acid is used in squashes. Acids increase the acidic content of food items, thus preventing the activity and growth of microorganisms.

- *Oils and spices:* Oils and spices are used as preservatives in pickles. Oils and spices prevent the growth of microorganisms, and spoilage is prevented. When pickle is made at home, the oil is poured to cover the mango, lemon or other vegetables which are used for making pickle. The oil acts as a protective cover and has two advantages:
  - prevents contact of microorganisms with the food, hence they cannot spoil the food.
  - prevents contact of air with food, hence the microorganisms cannot grow and spoil the food.

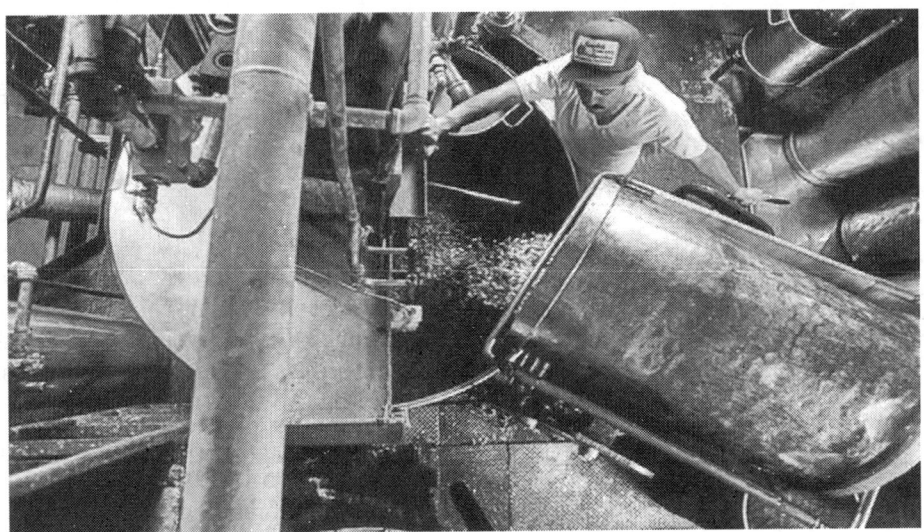

Canning at commercial level

2. Chemical Preservatives

Use of chemical preservatives:

- **Potassium metabisulphite:** Potassium metabisulfite preserves the natural color of food and protects food against bacteria.
- **Citric acid:** It is used as preservative in soft drinks.
- **Sodium benzoate:** Sodium benzoate is used for preventing molding. Sodium benzoate is commonly used in pickles, salad dressings, fruit juices, and soft drinks.

Canning

Canning is another important method of preserving the food items. Before canning the following steps are employed:

1. **Cleaning:** Cleaning is done for removing the dust and for removing the micro-organisms. At commercial level cleaning is done with the help of various kinds of washers. The raw materials may be subjected to high pressure sprays or strong flowing streams of water, while passing along a moving belt.

2. **Blanching:** Blanching consists of the immersion of raw food materials, especially vegetables and fruits, into hot water or exposure to live steam. Blanching serves as an additional hot water wash. It softens fibrous plant tissues, inhibits the action of enzymes and fixes the natural color of certain products making them more attractive in appearance.

3. **Exhausting:** Through this process gases are expelled by passing the open can containing the food through an exhaust box in which hot water or steam is used to expand the food and expel air and other gases from the contents and the head space area of the can. After expelling of the gases, the can is immediately sealed, heat processed and cooled.

4. **Sealing the container:** For avoiding the re-contamination the containers are sealed.

5. **Sterilization:** Sterilization is done for the prevention of spoilage from micro-organisms. This is usually done by the application of steam under pressure. The temperature and time used for heat processing depend on the kind of food, on the pH of the medium and other factors.

6. **Cooling:** After sterilization the containers are cooled to check the action of heat and

prevent unnecessary softening of the food or change in color of the contents. Cooling can be done by means of air or water.

Precautions during Preservation

Following are the precautions which are needed for preservation:

1. Proper care of hygiene should be taken during preparation and storage of food.

2. The utensils and containers used to cook and store food items should be thoroughly cleaned and dried in sun. The food items should be kept in air tight lids.

3. For preservation of pickles; all the vegetables or other items used during preparation should be covered with a layer of oil.

4. Clean and dried spoons are used while using the preserved food items.

5. The lid should be immediately closed after taking out the required quantity.

6. Bottles should be sterilized thoroughly before preserving the sauces and squashes.

Food Adulteration

Adulteration is defined as the process by which the quality of the given food item is reduced through the addition of a foreign or an inferior substance and the removal of a vital element.

TYPES OF ADULTERANTS

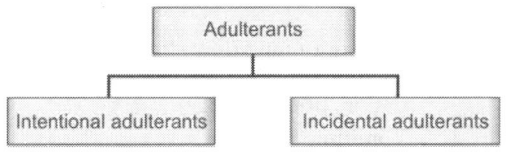

Intentional: Intentional adulterants are those substances that are added as a deliberate act on the part of the adulterer with the intention to increase the margin of profit. For example, sand, marble chips, stones, mud, chalk powder, water, dyes, etc. These adulterants cause harmful effects on the body.

Incidental: These adulterants are found in food substances due to ignorance, negligence or lack of proper facilities. It is not a willful act on the part of the adulterer. For example, pesticides, droppings of rodents, larvae in food.

Common food items, adulterants and health effect

S. No.	Adulterant	Foods commonly involved	Diseases or health effects
1.	Argemone seeds Argemone oil	Mustard seeds Edible oils and fats	Epidemic dropsy, glaucoma, cardiac arrest
2.	Artificially colored foreign seeds	As a substitute for cumin seed, poppy seed, black pepper	Injurious to health
3.	Foreign leaves or exhausted tea leaves, saw dust artificially colored	Tea	Injurious to health, cancer
4.	Tricresyl phosphate	Oils	Paralysis
5.	Rancid oil	Oils	Destroys vitamins A and E
6.	Sand, marble chips, stones, filth	Food grains, pulses, etc.	Damage digestive tract

(Contd.)

Common food items, adulterants and health effect (Contd.)

S. No.	Adulterant	Foods commonly involved	Diseases or health effects
7.	Lathyrus sativus	Khesari dal alone or mixed in other pulses	Lathyrism (crippling spastic paraplegia)
	Chemical contamination		
8.	Mineral oil (white oil, petroleum fractions)	Edible oils and fats, black pepper	Cancer
9.	Lead chromate	Turmeric whole and powdered, mixed spices	Anemia, abortion, paralysis, brain damage
10.	Methanol	Alcoholic liquors	Blurred vision, blindness, death
11.	Arsenic	Fruits such as apples sprayed over with lead arsenate	Dizziness, chills, cramps, paralysis, death
12.	Barium	Foods contaminated by rat poisons (barium carbonate)	Violent peristalsis, arterial hypertension, muscular twitching, convulsions, cardiac disturbances
13.	Cadmium	Fruit juices, soft drinks, etc. in contact with cadmium plated vessels or equipment. Cadmium contaminated water and shell-fish	'Itai-itai (ouch-ouch) disease, increased salivation, acute gastritis, liver and kidney damage, prostate cancer
14.	Cobalt	Water, liquors	Cardiac insufficiency and myocardial failure
15.	Lead	Water, natural and processed food	Lead poisoning (foot-drop, insomnia, anemia, constipation, mental retardation, brain damage)
16.	Copper	Food	Vomiting, diarrhea
17.	Tin	Food	Colic, vomiting
18.	Zinc	Food	Colic, vomiting
19.	Mercury	Mercury fungicide treated seed grains or mercury contaminated fish	Brain damage, paralysis, death

Common tests involved for detecting adulteration

S. No.	Food article	Adulteration	Test
1.	Vegetable oil	Castor oil	Take 1 ml of oil in a clean dry test tube. Add 10 ml of acidified petroleum ether. Shake vigorously for 2 minutes. Add 1 drop of ammonium molybdate reagent. The formation of turbidity indicates presence of castor oil in the sample.
		Argemone oil	Add 5 ml, conc. HNO_3 to 5 ml sample. Shake carefully. Allow to separate yellow, orange yellow, crimson color in the lower acid layer indicates adulteration.

(Contd.)

Common tests involved for detecting adulteration (*Contd.*)

S. No.	Food article	Adulteration	Test
2.	Ghee	Mashed potato, sweet potato, etc.	Boil 5 ml of the sample in a test tube. Cool and a drop of iodine solution. Blue color indicates presence of starch. Color disappears on boiling and reappears on cooling.
		Vanaspati	Take 5 ml of the sample in a test tube. Add 5 ml of hydrochloric acid and 0.4 ml of 2% furfural solution or sugar crystals. Insert the glass stopper and shake for 2 minutes. Development of a pink or red color indicates presence of vanaspati in ghee.
		Rancid stuff (old ghee)	Take one teaspoon of melted sample and 5 ml of HCl in a stoppered glass tube. Shake vigorously for 30 seconds. Add 5 ml of 0.1% of ether solution of phloroglucinol. Re-stopper and shake for 30 seconds and allow to stand for 10 minutes. A pink or red color in the lower (acid layer) indicates rancidity.
		Synthetic coloring matter	Pour 2 gm of filtered fat dissolved in ether. Divide into 2 portions. Add 1 ml of HCl to one tube. Add 1 ml of 10% NaOH to the other tube. Shake well and allow to stand. Presence of pink color in acidic solution or yellow color in alkaline solution indicates added coloring matter.
3.	Honey	Invert sugar/jaggery	1. Fiehe s test: Add 5 ml of solvent ether to 5 ml of honey. Shake well and decant the ether layer in a Petri dish. Evaporate completely by blowing the ether layer. Add 2 to 3 ml of resorcinol (1 gm of resorcinol resublimed in 5 ml of conc HCl.) Appearance of cherry red color indicates presence of sugar/jaggery.
			2. Aniline chloride test: Take 5 ml of honey in a porcelain dish. Add aniline chloride solution (3 ml of aniline and 7 ml of 1:3 HCl) and stir well. Orange red color indicates presence of sugar.
4.	Pulses/besan	Kesari dal (*Lathyrus sativus*)	Add 50 ml of dilute HCl to a small quantity of dal and keep on simmering water for about 15 minutes. The pink color, if developed indicates the presence of kesari dal.
5.	Pulses	Metanil yellow (dye)	Add conc HCl to a small quantity of dal in a little amount of water. Immediate development of pink color indicates the presence of metanil yellow and similar color dyes.

(Contd.)

Common tests involved for detecting adulteration (*Contd.*)

S. No.	Food article	Adulteration	Test
		Lead chromate	Shake 5 gm of pulse with 5 ml of water and add a few drops of HCl. Pink color indicates lead chromate.
6.	Bajra	Ergot infested bajra	Swollen and black ergot infested grains will turn light in weight and will float also in water.
7.	Wheat flour	Excessive sand and dirt	Shake a little quantity of sample with about 10 ml of carbon tetrachloride and allow to stand. Grit and sandy matter will collect at the bottom.
		Excessive bran	Sprinkle on water surface. Bran will float on the surface.
		Chalk powder	Shake sample with dilute HCl effervescence indicates chalk.
8.	Common spices like turmeric, chilly, curry powder, etc.	Color	Extract the sample with petroleum ether and add 13N H_2SO_4 to the extract. Appearance of red color (which persists even upon adding a little distilled water) indicates the presence of added colors. However, if the color disappears upon adding distilled water the sample is not adulterated.
9.	Black pepper	Papaya seeds/light berries, etc.	Pour the seeds in a beaker containing carbon tetrachloride. Black papaya seeds float on the top while the pure black pepper seeds settle down.
10.	Spices (ground)	Powdered bran and saw dust	Sprinkle on water surface. Powdered bran and sawdust float on the surface.
11.	Coriander powder	Dung powder	Soak in water. Dung will float and can be easily detected by its foul smell.
		Common salt	To 5 ml of sample add a few drops of silver nitrate. White precipitate indicates adulteration.
12.	Chillies	Brick powder grit, sand, dirt, filth, etc.	Pour the sample in a beaker containing, a mixture of chloroform and carbon tetrachloride. Brick powder and grit will settle at the bottom.
13.	*Badi elaichi* seeds	*Choti elaichi* seeds	Separate out the seeds by physical examination. The seeds of *badi elaichi* have nearly plain surface without wrinkles or streaks while seeds of cardamom have pitted or wrinkled ends.
14.	Turmeric powder	Starch of maize, wheat, tapioca, rice	A microscopic study reveals that only pure turmeric is yellow colored, big in size and has an angular structure. While foreign/added starches are colorless and small in size as compared to pure turmeric starch.

(Contd.)

Common tests involved for detecting adulteration (*Contd.*)

S. No.	Food article	Adulteration	Test
15.	Turmeric	Lead chromate	Ash the sample. Dissolve it in 1:7 sulphuric acid (H_2SO_4) and filter. Add 1 or 2 drops of 0.1% dipenylcarbazide. A pink color indicates presence of lead chromate.
		Metanil Yellow	Add a few drops of conc. hydrochloric acid (HCl) to sample. Instant appearance of violet color, which disappears on dilution with water, indicates pure turmeric. If color persists metanil yellow is present.
16.	Cumin seeds (black *jeera*)	Grass seeds colored with charcoal dust	Rub the cumin seeds on palms. If palms turn black adulteration in indicated.
17.	Asafoetida (*heeng*)	Soap stone, other earthy matter	Shake a little quantity of powdered sample with water. Soap stone or other earthy matter will settle at the bottom.
		Chalk	Shake sample with carbon tetrachloride (CCl_4). Asafoetida will settle down. Decant the top layer and add dilute HCl to the residue. Effervescence shows presence of chalk.
18.	Food grains	Hidden insect infestation	Take a filter paper impregnated with ninhydrin (1% in alcohol.) Put some grains on it and then fold the filter paper and crush the grains with hammer. Spots of bluish purple color indicate presence of hidden insects infestation.

Food Safety: Standards and Laws

Unhygienic and unsafe food causes many diseases, ranging from diarrheal diseases to various forms of other diseases. A safe and healthy food supply contributes to food and nutrition security, and stimulates sustainable development.

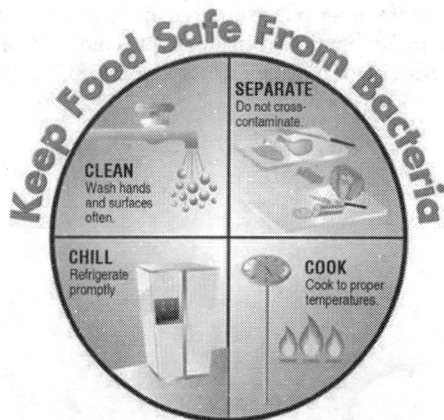

Food safety: The scientific discipline that deals with handling, preparation, and storage of food in ways through which food-borne illness is prevented. This includes a number of routines that should be followed to avoid potentially severe health hazards.

For ensuring the safety of food many systems are adopted.

The government has promulgated many laws and standards which protects the quality of food and ensures the supply of safe, nutritious and adulteration free food items.

INDIAN FOOD LAWS AND STANDARDS

1. ***Prevention of Food Adulteration Act, 1954:*** One of the early Acts to be promulgated was the Prevention of Food Adulteration (PFA) Act of 1954, which was in force since June 1, 1955. The objective of this act was to ensure that food articles sold to the consumers are pure and wholesome. The act prohibits the manufacture, sale and distribution of not only adulterated foods but also foods contaminated with microorganisms and toxicants. PFA specifies microbial safety standards for pasteurized milk, milk powder, skimmed milk powder, infant milk food, tomato sauce, jam, malted milk food and aflatoxin levels for groundnut. The PFA standards and regulations apply equally to domestic and imported products and cover various aspects of food processing and distribution. These include food colors, preservatives, pesticide residues, packaging and labeling and regulation of sales. 'A central committee for food standards' has been constituted under the Act and has been charged with the function of advising the central

the food standards. The state government sets up food testing laboratory and appoints public analysts with adequate staff to report on suspected foods.

2. *Fruit Products Order (1955):* The fruit and vegetable processing sector is regulated by the Fruit Products Order (FPO), 1955, which is administered by the department of food processing industries. The FPO contains specifications and quality control requirements regarding the production and marketing of processed fruits and vegetables, sweetened aerated water, vinegar and synthetic syrups. Packaging of fruits and vegetables of a standard below the minimum prescribed standards is an offence, punishable by law. All processing units are required to obtain a license under the FPO, and periodic inspections are carried out. Processed fruits and vegetable products imported into the country must meet the FPO standards.

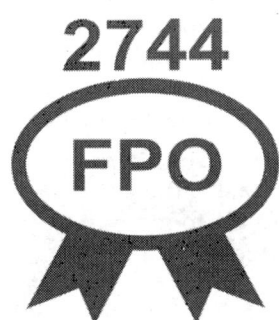

3. *Meat Products Order (1973):* The regulations made under the Act covers the meat products. The order:
   - Specifies sanitation and hygienic requirements for slaughter houses and manufacture of meat products.
   - Contains packing, marketing and labeling provisions for containers of meat products.
   - Defines the permissible quantity of heavy metals, preservatives and insecticide residues in meat products.
   - Prevents the use of harmful substances in meat food products. The directorate of marketing and inspection at the ministry of agriculture is the regulatory authority for the order, which is equally applicable to domestic processors and importers of meat products.

4. *Livestock Importation Act (1898):* India has established procedures for the importation of livestock under the Livestock Importation Act, 1898. Under the regulations, the import of meat products, eggs and egg powder and milk products require a sanitary import permit from the Department of Animal Husbandry, Dairying and Fisheries at the Ministry of Agriculture.

5. *Milk and Milk Products Order (1992):* Under milk and milk products order the production and distribution or supply of milk products is controlled by the Milk and Milk Products Order, 1992. The order sets sanitary requirements for dairies, machinery and premises and includes quality control, certification, packing, marketing and labeling standards for milk and milk products. Standards specified in the order also apply to imported products.

6. *Essential Commodities Act (1955):* The Act is mainly meant for regulating the manufacture, commerce and distribution of essential commodities including food to the public at reasonable price.

7. *Cold Storage Order (1980):* The Cold Storage Order, 1980, promulgated under the Essential Commodities Act, 1955, has the objective of earning hygienic and proper refrigeration conditions in a cold store regulating the growth of cold storage industry and rendering technical guidance for the scientific preservation of food stuffs in a cold store and prevent exploitation of farmers by cold store owners. Agricultural marketing advisor to the government of India is the licensing officer under this.

8. *Weights and Measures Act (1976):* Standards for weights and measures are

administered by the ministry of consumer affairs, food and public distribution under the Standards of Weights and Measures Act, 1976 and related Rules and notification. All weights or measures must be recorded in metric units and certain commodities can only be packed in specified quantities (weight, measure or number). These include baby and weaning foods, biscuits, bread, butter, coffee, tea, vegetable oils, milk powder, wheat, and rice flour.

9. *Consumer Protection Act (1986):* The Act came into effect first on December 24, 1986 after being passed by the Indian parliament. It was modified later on and the modifications came into effect on March 15, 2003. The Act makes provisions to include both tangible goods and intangible service purchased from trader or service provider. The main objective of this Act is to promote and protect the rights of the consumers, with regard to defective goods, deficiency of services, overcharging or any other unfair trade practices. Complaints can be referred to the district consumer redressal forum. The forum can order the opposite party for removal of the defect, replacement of the goods, return of the prices or charges or order payment of compensation for the loss or damage suffered due to deficiency of service. Appeals can be made to state commission and then to national commission.

Bureau of Indian Standards (BIS)

The Bureau of Indian Standards operates certification mark scheme under the BIS Act, 1986. Standards covering more than 450 different food products have been published. Standards are laid for vegetable and fruit products, spices and condiments, animal products and processed foods. Once these standards are accepted, manufacturers whose products confirm to these standards are allowed to use BIS label on each unit of their product. The products are checked for quality by the BIS testing laboratories at Delhi, Mumbai, Kolkata, Chennai, Chandigarh and Patna. Some of the items which require compulsory BIS certification under PFA are natural food colors and food color preparation, food additives, infant milk foods; milk cereal based weaning foods, milk powder and condensed milk.

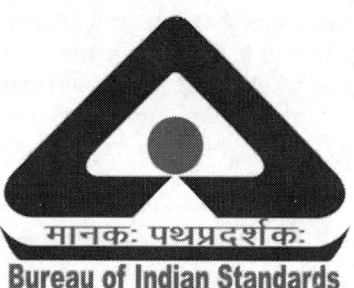

Bureau of Indian Standards

The AGMARK Standard

The word "AGMARK" is agricultural marketing. The AGMARK standard was set up by the directorate of marketing and inspection of the government of India by introducing an Agricultural Produce Act in 1937. The word "AGMARK" seal ensures quality and purity.

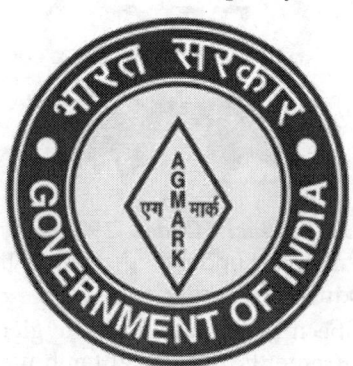

The Act defines quality of cereals, spices, oilseeds, oil, butter, ghee, legumes and eggs and provides for the categorization of commodities into various grades depending on the degree of purity in each case. The grades incorporated are grades 1, 2, 3 and 4 or special, good, fair and ordinary.

The central AGMARK laboratory at Nagpur continuously carries out research and development works in this field. The "certificate of authorization," is granted only to those in the trade having adequate experience and standing in the market.

Codex Alimentarius

The Codex Alimentarius Commission is an inter-governmental body was established in 1963. It has over 170-member countries within the framework of the joint FAO/WHO food standards programme established by the Food and Agriculture Organization of the United Nations (FAO) and the World Health Organization (WHO). Codex alimentarious sets guidelines and standards to ensure 'fair trade practices' and consumer protection in relation to the global trade of food. Its primary purpose is "protecting the health of consumers and ensuring fair practices in the food trade." The commission also promotes coordination of all food standards work undertaken by international governmental and non-governmental organizations (INGOs).

Consumer Disputes Redressal Agencies

This section of the act provides for the creation of consumer courts. The central government is given the responsibility to create and maintain the National Consumer Disputes Redressal Commission in New Delhi. The state government is given the responsibility to create a state consumer disputes redressal commission at the state level and a district consumer redressal forum at the district level. World consumer day is celebrated every year on 15th March.

Food Microbiology

Microbiology is the branch of the biological sciences that deals with microorganisms, i.e. bacteria, fungi, some algae, protozoa and viruses. Most microorganisms have the following characteristics:

I. They are generally too small to be seen with the unaided human eye, and some form of microscopy is required for the study of their structure.

II. Cells or other structures are relatively simple and less specialized than those of higher plants and animals.

III. They are handled and cultured in the laboratory in ways that are generally quite similar.

Food microbiology: The study of the role that microorganisms play in food spoilage, food production, food preservation and food-borne disease.

Food-borne diseases: Many pathogenic microorganisms (bacteria, molds and viruses) can contaminate foods during various stages of their handling, between production and consumption. Consumption of these foods can cause food-borne diseases. Food-borne diseases can be fatal and may also cause large economic losses. Foods of animal origin are associated with food-borne diseases.

Food spoilage: Except for sterile foods, all foods harbor microorganisms. Food spoilage stems from the growth of these micro-organisms in food or is due to the action of microbial enzymes. New marketing trends, consumers' desire for foods that are not overly processed and preserved, extended shelf life, and chances of temperature abuse between production and consumption of foods have greatly increased the chances of food spoilage, and in some instances, with new types of micro-organisms. The major concerns are the economic loss and wastage of food. New concepts are being studied to reduce contamination as well as control the growth of spoilage microbes in foods.

MICROORGANISMS IN FOOD

Molds are important in food because they can grow even in conditions in which many bacteria cannot grow, such as low pH, low water activity (Aw), and high osmotic pressure. Many types of molds are found in foods. They are important spoilage microorganisms. Many strains also produce mycotoxins and have been implicated in food-borne intoxication.

Some species or strains produce mycotoxins (e.g. *Aspergillus flavus* produces aflatoxin).

Many species or strains are also used in food and food additive processing. *Asp. oryzae* is used to hydrolyze starch by α-amylase in the production of sake. *Asp. niger* is used to process citric acid from sucrose and to produce enzymes such as β-galactosidase.

Alternaria. Members are septate and form dark-colored spores on conidia. They cause rot in tomatoes and rancid flavor in dairy products. Some species or strains produce mycotoxins. Species: *Alternaria tenuis.*

Fusarium. Many types are associated with rot in citrus fruits, potatoes, and grains. They form cottony growth and produce septate, sickle-shaped conidia. Species: *Fusarium solani.*

Mucor. It is widely distributed. Members have nonseptate hyphae and produce sporangiophores. They produce cottony colonies. Some species are used in food fermentation and as a source of enzymes. They cause spoilage of vegetables. Species: *Mucor rouxii.*

Penicillium. It is widely distributed and contains many species. Members have septate hyphae and form conidiophores on a blue-green, brushlike conidia head. Some species are used in food production, such as *Penicillium roqueforti* and *Pen. camemberti* in cheese. Many species cause fungal rot in fruits and vegetables. They also cause spoilage of grains, breads, and meat. Some strains produce mycotoxins (e.g. Ochratoxin A).

Rhizopus. Hyphae are aseptate and form sporangiophores in sporangium. They cause spoilage of many fruits and vegetables. *Rhizopus stolonifer* is the common black bread mold.

Important Yeast

Yeasts are important in food because of their ability to cause spoilage. Many are also used in food bioprocessing. Some are used to produce food additives.

Saccharomyces. Cells are round, oval, or elongated. It is the most important genus and contains heterogenous groups. *Saccharomyces cerevisiae* variants are used in baking for leavening bread and in alcoholic fermentation. They also cause spoilage of food, producing alcohol and CO_2.

Candida. Many species spoil foods with high acid, salt, and sugar and form pellicles on the surface of liquids. Some can cause rancidity in butter and dairy products (e.g. *Candida lipolytica*).

Zygosaccharomyces. Cause spoilage of high-acid foods, such as sauces, ketchups, pickles, mustards, mayonnaise, salad dressings, especially those with less acid and less salt and sugar (e.g., *Zygosaccharomyces bailii*).

Important Viruses

Viruses are important in food for three reasons. Some are able to cause enteric disease, and thus, if present in a food, can cause food-borne diseases. Hepatitis A viruses have been implicated in food-borne outbreaks. Several other enteric viruses, such as poliovirus, echo virus, and coxsackie virus, can cause food-borne diseases. In some countries where the level of sanitation is not very high, they can contaminate foods and cause disease.

Some bacterial viruses (bacteriophages) are used to identify some pathogens (*Salmonella* spp., *Staphylococcus aureus* strains) on the basis of the sensitivity of the cells to a series of bacteriophages at appropriate dilutions. Bacteriophages are used to transfer genetic traits in some bacterial species or strains by a process called transduction (e.g. in *Escherichia coli* or *Lactococcus lactis*).

Important Bacteria

A. **Lactic acid bacteria:** They are bacteria that produce relatively large quantities of lactic acid from carbohydrates. Species mainly from genera *Lactococcus, Leuconostoc, Pediococcus, Lactobacillus,* and *Streptococcus thermophilus* are included in this group.

B. Acetic acid bacteria: They are bacteria that produce acetic acid, such as *Acetobacter aceti.*

C. Propionic acid bacteria: They are bacteria that produce propionic acid and are used in dairy fermentation. Species such as *Propionibacterium freudenreichii,* etc. are included in this group.

D. Butyric acid bacteria: They are bacteria that produce butyric acid in relatively large amounts. Some *Clostridium* spp. such as *Clostridium butyricum* are included in this group.

E. Proteolytic bacteria: They are bacteria that can hydrolyze proteins because they produce extracellular proteinases. Species in genera *Micrococcus, Staphylococcus, Bacillus, Clostridium, Pseudomonas, Alteromonas, Flavobacterium, Alcaligenes,* some in *Enterobacteriaceae,* and *Brevibacterium* are included in this group.

F. Lipolytic bacteria: They are bacteria that are able to hydrolyze triglycerides because they produce extracellular lipases. Species in genera *Micrococcus, Staphylococcus, Pseudomonas, Alteromonas,* and *Flavobacterium* are included in this group.

G. Saccharolytic bacteria: They are bacteria that are able to hydrolyze complex carbohydrates. Species in genera *Bacillus, Clostridium, Aeromonas, Pseudomonas,* and *Enterobacter* are included in this group.

H. Thermophilic bacteria: They are bacteria that are able to grow at 50°C and above. Species from genera *Bacillus, Clostridium, Pediococcus, Streptococcus,* and *Lactobacillus* are included in this group.

I. Psychrotrophic bacteria: They are bacteria that are able to grow at refrigerated temperature. Some species from *Pseudomonas, Alteromonas, Alcaligenes, Flavobacterium, Serratia, Bacillus, Clostridium,* *Lactobacillus, Leuconostoc, Carnobacterium, Brochothrix, Listeria, Yersinia,* and *Aeromonas* are included in this group.

J. Gas-producing bacteria: They are bacteria that produce gas (CO_2, H_2, H_2S) during metabolism of nutrients. Species from genera *Leuconostoc, Lactobacillus, Propionibacterium, Escherichia, Enterobacter, Clostridium,* and *Desulfotomaculum* are included in this group.

K. Spore formers: They are bacteria having the ability to produce spores. Species from *Bacillus, Clostridium,* and *Desulfotomaculum* are included in this group. They are further divided into aerobic sporeformers, anaerobic sporeformers, flat sour sporeformers, thermophilic sporeformers, and sulfide-producing sporeformers.

L. Coliforms: Species from *Escherichia, Enterobacter, Citrobacter,* and *Klebsiella* are included in this group. They are used as an index of sanitation.

Factors Affecting Growth of Microorganisms

Temperature

Temperature is one of the important factor that control microbial growth. Based on their tolerance of broad temperature ranges, microorganisms are roughly classified as follows:

1. **Psychrophies:** Microorganisms grow only at refrigeration temperatures.

2. **Psychrotrophs:** Micoorganisms grow well at refrigeration temperatures, but better at room temperature.

3. **Mesophiles:** These microorganisms grow best at or near human body temperature, but grow well at room temperature.

4. **Thermophiles:** They grow only at temperatures about as hot as the human hand can endure, and usually not at all at or below body temperature.

Water activity: Water activity (a_w) is a term describing the availability of water to microorganisms.

pH: pH is a term used to describe the acidity or alkalinity of a solution. pH has a profound effect on the growth of microorganisms. Most bacteria grow best at about pH 7 and grow poorly or not at all below pH 4. Yeasts and molds, therefore, predominate in low pH foods where bacteria cannot compete. The lactic acid bacteria are exceptions; they can grow in high acid foods and actually produce acid to give us sour milk, pickles, fermented meats, and similar products. Some strains, called Leuconostoc contribute off-flavors to orange juice.

Oxygen: Oxygen is essential for growth of some microorganisms; these are called aerobes. Others cannot grow in its presence and are called anaerobes. Still others can grow either with or without oxygen and are called microaerophilic. Strict aerobes grow only on food surfaces and cannot grow in foods stored in cans or in other evacuated, hermetically sealed containers. Anaerobes grow only beneath the surface of foods or inside containers. Aerobic growth is faster than anaerobic. Therefore, in products where both conditions exist, such as in fresh meat, the surface growth is promptly evident, whereas subsurface growth is not.

MICROBIAL SPOILAGE OF FOOD

Fruits and fruit juices: Naturally fresh fruits and juices made out of them contain high amount of water thereby making them highly prone to attack by microorganisms.

Growth of lactic acid bacteria in juices and other fruit products cause the formation of haze, gas, acid, and a number of other changes. Certain heterofermentative lactobacilli lead to slime in cider.

Some strains of *Acetobacter pasteurianus* and *Gluconobacter oxydans* produce microfibrils composed of cellulose, which leads to formation of flocs in different fruit juice beverages.

Various spore formers such as *Bacillus coagulans, B. subtilis, B. macerans, B. pumilus, B. sphaericus, and B. pantothenticus* have been found to grow in different types of wines.

Cereals and its products: Most common species of molds are *Aspergillus, Rhizopus, Mucor, Fusarium.* A significant aspect of spoilage of molds is production of mycotoxins, which may pose danger to health.

Bread is a major product prepared using flours. Ropiness in bread is usually due to bacterial growth and is considered more prevalent in home made breads. The chief causative organism is *Bacillus subtilis* or *B. licheniformis.* These are spore forming bacteria with their spores surviving baking temperatures. These spores can germinate into vegetative cells, once they get suitable conditions as heat treatment activates them. In ropiness, the hydrolysis of bread flour protein (gluten) takes place by proteinases. Starch is also hydrolysed by amylases, which encourage ropiness. The manifestation of ropiness is development of yellow to brown color and soft and sticky surface. It is also accompanied by odor.

Vegetables

Bacterial Soft Rot

Caused by *Erwinia carotovora* and Pseudomonas such as *P. marginalis, Bacillus* and *Clostridium* spp. are also implicated.

Breaks down pectin, giving rise to a soft, mushy consistency, sometimes a bad odour and water-soaked appearance.

Vegetables affected—onions, garlic, beans, carrot, beets, lettuce, spinach, potatoes, cabbage, cauliflower, radishes, tomatoes, cucumbers, watermelons.

Fungal spoilage of vegetables

Penicillium, Cladosporium, Rhizopus, Aspergillus spp. are responsible for various defects in vegetables.

Spoilage of egg: The spoilage of eggs is caused by bacteria as compared to molds and can be described as green rot due to the growth of *Pseudomonas fluorescens*, colourless rot due to the growth of *Pseudomonas, Acinetobacter* and other species; black rots due to *P. roteus, Pseudomonas*; red rots due to *Serratia* spp. and custrad rots due to *Proteus vulgaris* and *P. intermedia.*

Growth of *Aeromonas* in the egg yolk turns it to black colour and also there is strong putrid odour due to the formation of hydrogen sulphide (H_2S).

Storage of eggs in high humid atmosphere may help in growth of several molds on the surface of the egg shell. Molds causing spoilage of eggs include species *of Pencillium, Mucor, Alterneria*, etc.

Spoilage of fish and sea foods: Halophilic bacteria like *Serratia, Micrococcus, Bacillus, Alcaligenes* and *Pseudomonas* cause spoilage of salt fish.

Shell fish are spoiled by *Acenetobacter, Moraxella* and *Vibrio*. Crab meat is spoiled by *Pseudomonas, Acinetobacter* and *Moraxella* at low temperature and by *Proteus* at high temperature.

Microbial loads in shrimps, oysters, and clams depend on the quality of the water from which they are harvested. If the sewage is drained to water bodies, the microbial quality deteriorates. During handling, fecal coliforms, fecal streptococci, and *S. aureus* may be incorporated into the product. *Salmonella* also is found in oysters possibly due to contaminated water.

Seafood also is the source for *Pseudomonas* spp., *C. perfringens, L. monocytogenes, Vibrio parahaemolyticus, Salmonella enterica serovar enteritidis* and *typhimurium, Campylobacter*

jejuni, Yersinia enterocolitica, and Enteroviruses (hepatitis A).

Smoked salmon and shrimps also are found to carry pathogenic *L. monocytogenes*.

Meat and Meat Products

Clostridium spp. are associated with spoilage of vacuum-packaged meats.

Change in colour of meat pigment: The red colour of meat may be changed to shades of green, brown or grey by *Lactobacillus* and *Leconostocs* spp.

Changes in fat: The unsaturated fat in meat gets oxidized by lypolitic bacteria which produce off odours due to hydrolysis of fats and production of aldehydes and acids. This type of spoilage is caused by lypolitic *Pseudomonas*, Achromobacter and yeast.

Actinomycetes produce musty or earthy flavor. Yeast also cause sliminess discoloration and off odor and taste defects.

Spoilage of milk: Milk is the best source of calcium and, what's more, it contains sodium, magnesium, potassium, zinc, carotene, protein, vitamins and essential amino acids. Milk substitutes such as soy, rice or almond milk usually contain much fewer nutrients.

Contamination in milk occurs due to poor hygiene. Some of the microorganisms responsible for spoilage of milk are as follows:

a. **Salmonella:** Salmonella are among the main causes of food poisoning. Salmonella are killed by pasteurization; raw milk and dried milk products are vulnerable.

b. **Listeria:** Contaminations with *Listeria monocytogenes* have been a major problem for the dairy industry recently.

c. **E. coli:** Certain species of the bacterium *E. coli* produce shigatoxin which may cause symptoms like diarrhea and stomach pain, sometimes even leading to life-threatening complications like hemolytic-uremic syndrome. *E. coli* are killed by pasteurization, infections due to milk products occur time and again.

d. **Pseudomonas**: The species *Pseudomonas fluorescens* is among the most common spoilage agents in milk. The enzymes produced by Pseudomonas are heat-stable and can survive pasteurization.

e. **Bacillus cereus**: The bacterium *Bacillus cereus* causes spoilage of cream, cheese and milk and makes them taste rancid, sour or bitter. *Bacillus cereus* produces toxins which may cause serious gastrointestinal disorders.

f. **Clostridium**: Clostridia form heat-resistant spores which can survive pasteurization at least partially. The species *Clostridium tyrobutyricum* is particularly feared in dairy production, because it causes so-called late blowing in raw milk cheese.

g. **Campylobacter**: *Campylobacter*, especially the species *C. jejuni*, is one of the main causes of food-borne diarrheal diseases.

Food Waste and its Management

Food waste is a biodegradable waste discharged from various sources including food processing industries, households, and hospitality sector. According to FAO, nearly 1.3 billion tonnes of food including fresh vegetables, fruits, meat, bakery, and dairy products are lost along the food supply chain. The amount of food waste has been projected to increase in the next 25 years due to economic and population growth. This food waste, which is a component of municipal solid waste, is incinerated or dumped in open area which may cause severe health and environmental issues.

Incineration of food waste consisting high moisture content results in the release of dioxins which may further lead to several environmental problems. Therefore, appropriate methods are required for the management of food waste.

Composition

Food waste mainly consists of carbohydrates, proteins, lipids, and traces of inorganic compounds. The composition varies in accordance with the type of food waste and its constituents. Food waste consisting of rice and vegetables is abundant in carbohydrates while food waste consisting of meat and eggs has high quantity of proteins and lipids.

MANAGEMENT

Planning

Planning carefully for grocery shopping is an effective tool to prevent overbuying, and consequently, food waste. Before going to market it is necessary to know which meal is planned and for how many members meal have to be prepared.

Purchasing

Purchasing accurate amount of food is essential for preventing food from wastage. It is essential to follow a routine of buying the food actually needed.

Storing

Proper storage and categorization of food products in combination with periodic re-ordering can lower food waste generation. During processes of ordering and disposal, food items can be re-examined, re-experienced, and re-valued, e.g. to be used for a meal, replaced within the place of storage, or moved out of it

Cooking

Too much food prepared ends up with being thrown away. A greater frequency of cooking is likely to enhance cooking skills such as more precise portion control. A better estimation of portion sizes is one of the most promising factor of avoiding food wastage. Another effective waste prevention strategy is cooking based on what is stored at home should be cooked first then further planning for cooking should be done.

Managing leftovers

One of the important strategies for preventing food wastage is reusing leftovers. Those who regularly eat leftovers produce less food waste.

Disposal/redistribution

The way in which food is disposed of also influences the amount of food wasted. Considerable amounts of food waste are given to pets. A focus on disposal practices, such as recycling or composting, often undermines people's motivation for waste prevention.

Redistribution of surplus food is scarce. Gifting and giving the food among close family members or to some person who is in need of food can be effective in combating the problem of food wastage.

Retailer options

Retailers can support the reduction of food waste by avoiding bulk purchases or by selling less aesthetic foods at discounts.

Conclusion

Proper planning, purchasing, cooking and distribution of food can prevent food wastage and can save the environment also. However, difficulties accompanying the collection as well as transportation of food waste should also be considered. The creation of favourable framework conditions as well as the support and cooperation with stakeholders along the supply chain are of utmost importance for a more sustainable and appreciative handling of food.

Applications of Nanotechnology in Nutrition

Nanotechnology is a field of research and innovation concerned with building 'things'—generally, materials and devices—on the scale of atoms and molecules.

According to Webster's Dictionary Nanotechnology is *"the manipulation of materials on an atomic or molecular scale especially to build microscopic devices"*.

Recent innovations in nanotechnology have transformed a number of scientific and industrial areas including the food industry. Advances in nutritional applications of nanotechnology include enhanced nutritional quality and flavor of food, bacterial growth detection, detection of food-borne pathogens, and polymer coatings applied to increase shelf-life of produce. Biomedical advances with nutritional implications include development of medical devices that helps in disease detection, and drug delivery systems are designed to target specific tissues.

Applications of nanotechnology have emerged with increasing need of nanoparticle uses in various fields of food science and food microbiology, including food processing, food packaging, functional food development, food safety, detection of food-borne pathogens, and shelf-life extension of food and/or food products.

Nanotechnology and increase in shelf-life of products: Nanotechnology is playing a important role in increasing the shelf-life of different kinds of food materials and also help brought down the extent of wastage of food due to microbial infestation.

Nanotechnology and food quality: Nanotechnology provides a range of options to improve the food quality and also helps in enhancing food taste.

Food packaging and nanotechnology: A desirable packaging material must have gas and moisture permeability combined with strength and biodegradability. Nano-based "smart" and "active" food packaging confer several advantages over conventional packaging methods from providing better packaging material with improved mechanical strength, barrier properties, antimicrobial films to nanosensing for pathogen detection and alerting consumers to the safety status of food.

Nanotechnology in agriculture: Nanotechnology will revolutionize agriculture and food industry by innovation new techniques such as precision farming techniques, enhancing the ability of plants to absorb nutrients, more efficient and targeted use of inputs, disease detection and control diseases, withstand environmental pressures and effective systems for processing, storage and packaging.

Nanotechnology in diagnosis of diseases: Nanotechnology is being studied for both the diagnosis and treatment of diseases such as atherosclerosis, or the build-up of plaque in arteries. In one technique, researchers created a nanoparticle that mimics the body's "good" cholesterol, known as HDL (high-density lipoprotein), which helps to shrink plaque.

Nanomedicine researchers are looking ways that nanotechnology can improve vaccines and developing various new medicines for the treatment of cancer.

Role of nanotechnology in food safety: Nanotechnology also have a big role in safety issues. Through nanotechnology the microbial contaminants are identified and toxin detection, shelf-life, and packaging strategies are improved. In addition, nanomaterials, including metal nanoparticles, carbon nanotubes, and other active nanomaterials can be used to develop biosensors for knowing the number of microbes present and other tests for food safety applications.

Nutraceuticals and nanotechnology: Nutraceuticals are defined as components or the nutrients that are isolated from foods and have health benefits besides providing nutrition and are therefore helps in preventing the occurrence of a disease.

Nowadays principle of nanotechnology has been utilized by researchers for the efficient delivery of these nutraceuticals with the aim to enhance their biological activity. A number of formulation approaches like nano-emulsions, micelles, nanoparticles, nanocapsules, etc. have been utilized for the efficient delivery of the encapsulated nutraceutical.

Nutraceuticals

Nutraceutical= 'Nutrition' + 'Pharmaceutical'. Nutraceuticals are food or part of food which are playing a major role in maintaining normal physiological functions of the body and thus are helping in managing various health problems. The principal reasons for the growth of the nutraceuticals worldwide are the current health problems developing in population and the health trends. Nutraceuticals have led to the new era of medicine and health. The new lifestyle today has changed the basic food habits and consumption of the junk food has increased which have lead to the number of diseases like obesity, cardiovascular diseases, cancer and other diseases. Obesity and heart disease continues to be a primary cause of death in most of the developing countries worldwide, followed by other diseases. Consumers due to expensive treatment are now focusing on alternative having natural and inexpensive aspects with beneficial effects on health.

Nutraceutical is defined as a food or part of a food that allegedly provides medicinal or health benefits, including the prevention and treatment of disease. A nutraceutical may be a naturally nutrient-rich or medicinally active food.

According to Dr. DeFelice Nutraceutical is defined as *"A food, or part of a food, that provides medical or health benefits, including the prevention and/or treatment of a disease."*

Health Benefits of Nutraceuticals

The health benefits of nutraceuticals has been combined with the treatment of many disorders such as metabolic problems, cancer, depression, diabetes, delayed gastric emptying time coronary artery disease and other health problems which needs care.

The common health benefits of nutraceuticals are as follows:

- They do not have any side effects.
- They have beneficial effect on health.
- Improves health.

Classification of Nutraceuticals

The food products used as nutraceuticals can be categorized as dietary fibre, prebiotics, probiotics, polyunsaturated fatty acids, antioxidants and other different types of herbal/natural foods. These nutraceuticals help in combating some of the major health problems of the century such as obesity, cardiovascular diseases, cancer, osteoporosis, arthritis, diabetes, cholesterol, etc.

Nutraceuticals or functional foods can be classified on the basis of their natural sources, pharmacological conditions, or as per chemical constitution of the products.

Nutraceuticals are classified as:

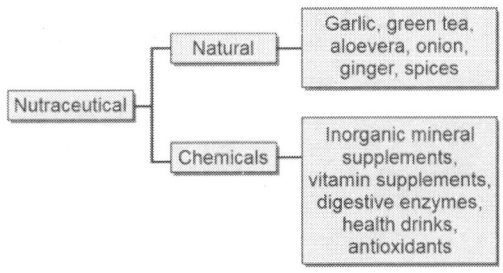

Natural products have been known for their therapeutic values for centuries. In the modern era, these substances have been used as an immunity booster; antidiabetic, anticancer, antimicrobial, and gastroprotective agents; and so on. Therefore, natural products could be better options to be formulated as nutraceuticals. Nutraceuticals have proven health benefits and their consumption that allow humans to maintain an overall good health. Nutraceuticals are the best way that helps maintaining health without side effects and acts against various health diseases with promoting optimal health, longevity, and quality of life.

Therapeutic Nutrition

Therapeutic diets are foods which are given in modified form during the special conditions of lifestyle changes that have strict parameters and a narrow focus. The intention of a diet of this sort is to cleanse, build or increase health following severe illness. Some therapeutic diets could result in vitamin and mineral deficiencies. There are many sustainable, healthy diets that produce holistic results to offset severe illnesses.

Another factor to be considered while planning for therapeutic diet is the diet history. The diet history of the patients help in revealing the patient's past food habits and also his likes and dislikes. The hours of the meal and the economic feasibility should also be considered.

Principles of Therapeutic Diet

The most important principle is to provide all the necessary nutrients so that a good nutritional status is achieved. In the diseased condition, the tissues become weak due to inadequacy of nutrients and the essential nutrients are also not utilized. Due to poor utilization of nutrients the digestion becomes difficult and the transportation of nutrients and absorption of the nutrients are also hampered, thus the nutritional status is also hampered.

Thus, the diet should be nutritionally adequate and should be modified in such a way that the recovery of the affected part occurs readily and the nutritional requirements of the individual are also met.

Objectives of Diet Therapy

The main objectives of diet therapy are:
1. To maintain good nutritional status.
2. To correct nutrient deficiencies which have occurred due to the disease.
3. To afford rest to the whole body or to the specific organ affected by the disease.
4. To adjust the food intake to the body's ability to metabolize the nutrients during the disease.
5. To bring about changes in body weight whenever necessary.

The advantages of therapeutic diets are:
• Psychological needs are fulfilled.
• Easy way of improving nutritional status.
• Nutritional values are obtained.
• All the essential factors of the diet can be included.

THERAPEUTIC DIETS

Routine Hospital Diets

1. *Clear liquid diet:* Clear liquid diet is diet without residue and served in fluid form. The diet is non-stimulating, non-irritating and does not form gas. The diet is served in small amounts (usually 30–60 ml) at frequent intervals (2 hours) to replace fluid and electrolytes and to relieve thirst. The diet is mainly composed of water, carbohydrates and some electrolytes provide only 400–500 kcal, 5 g protein, no fat. Clear liquid diet nutritionally inadequate and therefore, used for a very short period of time.

   Disease conditions in which the diet are used:
   i. Preoperative patients.
   ii. Postoperative patients, e.g. in the initial recovery phase after abdominal surgery or after a period of intravenous feeding.
   iii. Endoscopy or colonic examination.
   iv. Acute illness and infections.
   v. As the first step in oral alimentation of a nutritionally debilitated person.
   vi. Temporary food intolerance.
   vii. During diarrhea or to relieve thirst.
   viii. For reducing of colonic fecal matter.

2. *Full fluid diet:* Full fluid diet mainly includes the diet which is liquid and is adequately nutritious for patients who cannot chew or who are too ill to do so. It is free from cellulose and irritating condiments and spices. The diet should not be followed for more than two days. This diet is given in between a clear liquid diet and soft diet. The diet provides about 1200 kcal of energy and 35 g of protein. This should be given at 2–4 hour interval.

   Disease conditions in which the diet are given:
   i. Most often used postoperatively by patients progressing from clear liquids to solid foods.
   ii. During acute gastritis and infections.
   iii. Oral surgery or plastic surgery of face or neck area.
   iv. Chewing and swallowing dysfunction for acutely ill patients.
   v. Esophageal or stomach disorder who cannot tolerate solid foods owing to anatomical irregularity.

3. *Soft diet:* A soft diet is used as a transitional diet between full fluid and normal diet. Soft diet is nutritionally adequate. Soft diet is given in the form of soft food which is seasoned lightly. It is soft in consistency, easy to chew, made up of simple, easily digested foods, containing limited fiber and connecting tissues and does not contain rich or highly flavored foods. The soft diet supplies around 1800 kcal and 50 g protein.

   Disease conditions in which the diet are used:
   i. Postoperative patients who are unable to tolerate general diet.
   ii. Patients with mild GI problems.
   iii. Weak patients or patients with inadequate dentition to handle all foods in a general diet.
   iv. Diarrhea convalescence.

4. *Mechanical soft diet:* Mechanical diets are prescribed for the people who have lost their teeth. In this diet all the food items in a minced or chopped form can be given.

   Disease conditions for its use:
   i. Patients who are unable to chew.
   ii. Patients who have undergone head and neck surgery.
   iii. Dental problems.
   iv. Anatomical esophageal strictures.

5. *Normal diet:* A normal diet consists of any and all foods eaten by a person in good health. The diet is planned by including all the basic food groups in diet so that

optimum amounts of all nutrients are provided. The diet is well balanced and nutritionally adequate. The diet includes the careful attention of dietitian to monitor the food selection and food intake. The RDAs are taken into consideration to achieve the nutritional adequacy. Since the patient is hospitalized or is at bed rest, a reduction and the addition of the nutrients depend on the condition of the patients. The proteins are slightly increased to counteract a negative nitrogen balance. All other nutrients are supplied in normal amounts.

6. *Semi-liquid diets:* This diet is given following tonsillectomy or throat surgery until a soft or general diet may be swallowed without difficulty. It contains cold beverages and lukewarm preparations.

7. *Blenderized liquid diet:* The food items are given in blenderized form and it is given during oral surgery.

SPECIAL FEEDING METHODS

The different modes of feeding patients are:

Enteral

Enteral mode of feeding means, "within or by the way of the gastrointestinal tract." The foods are administered via tube and enteral feeding is also called tube feeding.

Tube Feeding

Tube feeding may be advised where the patient is unable to eat but the digestive system is functioning normally. Full fluid diets or commercial formulas may be administered through this route.

Different Modes of Tube Feeding

These are:

1. *Nasogastric tube feeding:* When the tube is passed through the nose into the stomach.

2. *Nasoduodenal tube feeding:* When the tube is passed through the nose into the duodenum.

3. *Nasojejunal tube feeding:* When tube is passed through the nose into jejunum. When there is an obstruction in the esophagus, enteral feeding is done by passing tube surgically through an incision in the abdominal wall into the stomach (gastrostomy), duodenum (duodenostomy) or jejunum (jejunostomy).

Conditions for Tube Feeding

1. Inability to swallow due to paralysis of muscles of swallowing (diphtheria, poliomyelitis).

2. Unwillingness to eat.

3. Persistent anorexia requiring forced feeding.

4. Semiconscious or unconscious patients.

5. Severe malabsorption requiring administration of unpalatable formula.

6. Short bowel syndrome.

7. Low birth weight babies.

Parenteral Nutrition

In parenteral nutrition, nutrients are delivered directly into the circulation through the peripheral or central vein is termed as parenteral nutrition. Intravenous feeding done in conditions when the patient cannot eat, will not eat, should not eat, cannot eat enough or cannot be fed adequately by tube feeding.

Conditions during which parenteral nutritional occur are:

1. Cancer

2. Inflammatory bowel disease

3. Short-bowel syndrome

4. Preoperative patients

5. Gastrointestinal disorders

Parenteral Feed Formula

The parenteral feed solutions contain:

- Glucose
- Emulsified fat
- Crystalline amino acids
- Vitamins
- Electrolytes—sodium, chlorine, phosphorus, potassium, calcium and magnesium.
- Trace elements—zinc, copper, chromium, manganese and iodine
- Water

Advantages of enteral feeding over intravenous feeding:

1. This is a convenient method of administration of nutrients.
2. It is inexpensive.
3. Easily tolerated.
4. No chances of metabolic disturbance.

Technology of Vegetable Products

India's favorable agro-climatic condition produces a variety of vegetables. The annual production of these crops is about 53 million tonnes.

Vegetables are plants or parts of plants served with the main course of a meal. Apart from the nutritive value, vegetables play important role in diet. They add appetizing color, texture and flavor to our daily food. With the wide choice of color of vegetables, it is possible to select a vegetable with a desired color to increase the appearance of a meal.

The texture of a vegetable varies depending upon whether it is served raw are cooked. The texture and appearance of meals can then be varied by the way the vegetable is served.

Vegetables contain a wide range of characteristic flavors. By a proper choice of vegetables, the desired flavor of a meal can be obtained.

▌ CLASSIFICATION OF VEGETABLES

Vegetables can be classified into three groups according to their nutritive value.

- Green leafy vegetables
- Roots and tubers
- Other vegetables

▌ GENERAL PROPERTIES OF VEGETABLES

Vegetables are derived from various parts of plants and it is sometimes useful to associate different vegetables with the parts of the plant they represent since this provides clues to some of the characteristics we may expect in these items. A classification of vegetables based on morphological features is given below.

Table: Classification of vegetables

Category	Examples
Vegetables, roots	Sweet potatoes, carrots
Stems tubers	Potatoes
Bulbs	Onions, garlic
Green leafy vegetables	
Leaves	Cabbage, spinach, lettuce
Flower buds	Cauliflower
Sprouts, shoots (young stems)	Asparagus, bamboo shoots
Fruit vegetables	
Legumes	Peas, green beans
Cereals	Sweet corn
Vine fruits	Squash, cucumber
Berry fruits	Tomato, egg plant
Tree fruits	Avocado, breadfruit

NUTRITIONAL COMPOSITION

Nutritional compositions of vegetables vary for a given kind in according to botanical variety, cultivation practices, and weather. It also varies with the change with maturity prior to harvest, and the condition of ripeness. Nutritional composition is also influenced by storage conditions.

Most fresh vegetables are high in water content, low in protein, and low in fat. In these cases water contents will generally be greater than 70% and frequently greater than 85%.

Legumes such as peas and certain beans are higher in protein; a few vegetables such as sweet corn which are slightly higher in fat and avocados which are substantially higher in fat.

Vegetables are important sources of both digestible and indigestible carbohydrates. The digestible carbohydrates are present largely in the form of sugars and starches while indigestible cellulose provides roughage which is important to normal digestion.

Vegetables are also important sources of minerals and certain vitamins, especially vitamins A and C.

The precursors of vitamin A, including beta-carotene and certain other carotenoids, are present in the yellow-orange vegetables and in some green leafy vegetables.

Potatoes also provide an important source of vitamin C for the diets.

Mineral Substances

Vegetables are good sources of minerals. The mineral content of vegetables varies normally between 0.60 and 1.80%.

The major elements are: Potassium (K), Sodium (Na), Calcium (Ca), Magnesium (Mg), Iron (Fe), Manganese (Mn), Aluminium (Al), Phosphorus (P), Chlorine (Cl), Sulphur (S).

Among the vegetables which are especially rich in mineral substances are:

- Spinach
- Carrots
- Cabbage
- Tomatoes, etc.

Vegetables usually contain more calcium than fruit; green beans, cabbage, onions and beans contain more than 0.1% calcium.

The calcium/phosphorus or Ca/P ratio is essential for calcium fixation in the human body. The adequate proportion of calcium and phosphorus is considered important for adults and children.

Carbohydrates

Carbohydrates are the main component of diet and are major source of energy. Carbohydrates play a major role in biological systems and in foods. Carbohydrates serve as structural components as in the case of cellulose; they may be stored as energy reserves as in the case of starch in plants.

Carbohydrates can be oxidized to furnish energy, and glucose in the blood is a ready source of energy for the human body. Carbohydrates after fermentation by yeast and other microorganisms can yield carbon dioxide, alcohol, organic acids and other compounds.

Important property of starches:

- Starch acts as reserve energy source.

Important properties of celluloses and hemicelluloses:

- These are important form of carbohydrates and are found abundantly in plant foods and act primarily as supporting structures in the plant tissues;
- They are insoluble in cold and hot water;
- They are not digested by man and so do not yield energy for nutrition;
- The fiber in food which produces necessary roughage is largely cellulose.

Important properties of pectins and carbohydrate gums.

- Pectins are common in fruits and vegetables and are gum-like substances (they are found in and between cell walls) and helps in holding the plant cells together;

- Pectins in colloidal solution contribute to viscosity of the tomato paste;
- Pectins in solution form gels when sugar and acid are added; and
- Pectin is the basis of jelly manufacture.

Fats

Vegetables contain very low level of fats.

Nitrogen-containing Substances

These substances are found in plants as different combinations: Proteins, amino acids, amides, amines, nitrates, etc. Among nitrogen containing substances the most important are proteins; they have a colloidal structure and, by heating, their water solution above 50°C an one-way reaction makes them insoluble. This behavior has to be taken into account in heat processing of vegetables.

Vitamins

Basically there are two types of vitamins:

A. *Fat-soluble vitamins:* These include vitamins A, D, E and K. Their absorption by the body depends upon the normal absorption of fat from the diet.

B. *Water-soluble vitamins:* These include vitamin C and several members of the vitamin B complex. Vegetables are good sources of water soluble vitamins.

Vitamin A (Retinol)

Vitamin A: Sources are meat, milk, eggs and all yellow fruits and vegetables.

Plant foods contain no vitamin A but contain its precursor, beta-carotene. Human being requires either vitamin A or beta-carotene which can be easily converted to vitamin A in the body.

All the yellow vegetables are good sources of beta-carotene. Vegetables such as potatoes, pumpkin, spinach are good sources of beta-carotene.

Vitamin C (Ascorbic Acid)

Vitamin C readily destroyed by oxidation especially at high temperatures. Vitamin C is easily lost during processing, storage and cooking.

All the citrus fruits are excellent sources of vitamin C. Vegetables such as tomatoes, cabbage and green peppers are good sources of vitamin C.

Potatoes also are a fair source (content of vitamin C is low) of vitamin C.

Enzymes

Enzymes are biological catalysts that promote most of the biochemical reactions which occur in vegetable cells.

Some properties of enzymes important in vegetable technology are the following:

- Enzymes are required for ripening of vegetables.
- Enzymes play an important role in various biochemical reactions of the vegetables.
- Enzymes are important for color, flavor and textures of vegetables.

Texture

The range of textures that are encountered in cooked vegetables is indeed great, and to a large extent can be explained in terms of changes in specific cellular components.

The texture of vegetable food items varies and changes upon cooking.

Sources of Color and Change in Color after Cooking

Color plays an important role in food acceptance. The color in vegetables creates interest and makes food appealing and thus increases its acceptability.

The compounds which are responsible for color in vegetables are called pigments.

These pigments are classified into four major groups:

1. Chlorophylls
2. Carotenoids
3. Anthocyanins
4. Anthoxanthins.

The chlorophylls: The chlorophylls are contained mainly within the chloroplasts and have a primary role in the photosynthetic production of carbohydrates from carbon dioxide and water. The bright green color of leaves and other parts of plants is largely due to the oil-soluble chlorophylls, which in nature are bound to protein molecules in highly organized complexes.

Points to Remember

- Cooking leads to change in color. After cooking chlorophyll changes to pheophytin. The color changes from olive green to brown.

- Conversion to pheophytin is favored by acid pH but does not occur readily under alkaline conditions. For these reason peas, beans, spinach, and other green vegetables which tend to lose their bright green colors on heating can be largely protected against such color changes by the addition of sodium bicarbonate or other alkali to the cooking or canning water.

In food processing the carotenoids are fairly resistant to heat, changes in pH, and water leaching since they are fat-soluble. However, they are very sensitive to oxidation, which results in both color loss and destruction of vitamin A activity.

Flavonoids: The flavonoids include the purple, blue, and red anthocyanins of grapes, berries, plump, eggplant, and cherry; the yellow anthoxanthins of light colored fruit and vegetables such as apple, onion, potato, and cauliflower, and the colorless catechins and leuco-anthocyanins which are food tannins and are found in apples, grapes, tea, and other plant tissues. These colorless tannin compounds are easily converted to brown pigments upon reaction with metal ions.

Properties of the anthocyanins include a shifting of colors with pH. Thus, many of the anthocyanins which are violet or blue in alkaline media become red upon addition of acid.

Cooking of beets with vinegar tends to shift the color from a purplish red to a brighter red, while alkaline water can influence the color of red fruits and vegetables toward violet and gray-blue.

The anthocyanins also tend toward the violet and blue hues upon reaction with metal ions, which is one reason for lacquering the inside of metal cans when the true color of anthocyanin-containing fruits and vegetables is to be preserved.

The water-soluble property of anthocyanins also results in easy leaching of these pigments from cut fruit and vegetables during processing and cooking.

The yellow anthoxanthins also are pH sensitive tending toward a deeper yellow in alkaline media. Thus, potatoes or apples become somewhat yellow when cooked in water with a pH of 8 or higher, which is common in many areas. Acidification of the water to pH 6 or lower favors a whiter color.

The colorless tannin compounds upon reaction with metal ions form a range of dark colored complexes which may be red, brown, green, grey, or black. The various shades of these colored complexes depend upon the particular tannin, the specific metal ion, pH, concentration of the complex, and other factors not yet fully understood.

NEED FOR INCLUSION OF VEGE-TABLES IN DIET

1. Vegetables provide vitamins and minerals required for growth and maintenance of health and are thus termed as protective foods.

2. Roots and tubers provide energy.

3. Vegetables are low in fat and can be used liberally in low calorie diets for weight reduction.

4. Besides providing nutrients they add variety to the diet. They make the diet attractive by their texture, flavor and color.

5. Vegetables contain phytochemicals. The term phytochemicals refers to the wide variety of plant compounds naturally produced by plants. They include plant pigments and flavoring substances. Vegetables with bright colors, viz. yellow, orange, red, green, blue, purple contain phytochemicals.

6. Beta-carotene, vitamin C and vitamin E are nutrients that function as antioxidants. An antioxidant is a substance that significantly reduces or prevents oxidation of fatty acids and protein thus preventing cell and tissue damage caused by free radicals in the body. These free radicals attack healthy cells in the body which leads to degeneration of cells.

Intake of fibrous vegetables are important as they:

- Give satiety and thereby decrease food intake.
- Help in regulating bowel movement.
- Low in calorie content.
- Reduce blood cholesterol levels.
- Promote chewing and decrease rate of ingestion.

7. Vegetables are used in the preparation of salads.

PRODUCTS PREPARED FROM VEGETABLES

Vegetables plays important role in preparation of various food items. These products are popular in various regions and add variety and flavor in the diet. There are hundreds of varieties in existence and they can be made from a wide range of fruits and vegetables.

There are various items which are prepared from vegetable. These items are prepared and then preserved so that they can be enjoyed in different seasons. The food items are preserved by adding various preservatives.

For example: Acetic acid preserves the product by making the environment acidic, and this inhibits the growth of spoilage and food-poisoning microorganisms. Other ingredients such as salt and sugar add to the preservative effect.

Vegetable Products

Chutney

These are jam-like mixtures which have added vinegar and spices. The high sugar content exerts a preservative effect, and a high level

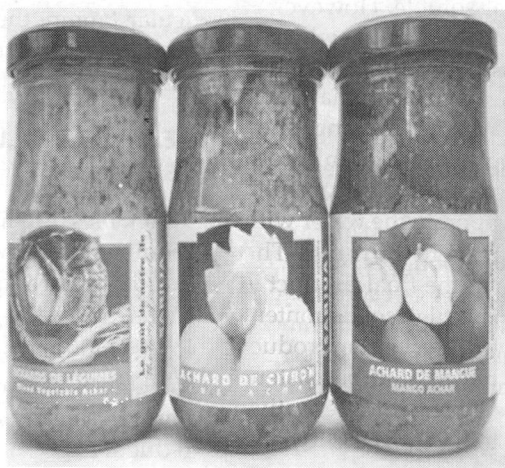

of vinegar addition is not always needed. These products are hot-filled.

Pickles

Pickles are prepared at household level and also at commercial level. For the preparation of pickles the vegetables are first chopped and then they are mixed with various spices and salt, these are preserved in oils or in vinegar. Pickles can be fermented or unfermented, sweet or sour, and can be made from either whole or chopped fruit.

Sauces

Sauces are thick liquids made from pulped fruit and/or vegetables, with the addition of salt, spices, sugar, and vinegar. They require pasteurization and are filled while hot.

Soups

Soups are also prepared with vegetables. The food which is to be used for making soup is cooked thoroughly in plenty of water. Clear soups are prepared using only the water in which the vegetable is cooked. Soups provide us with a variety of nutrients depending on the ingredients used. Soups also enhance appetite and add color to the meal. It is usually served at the beginning of a meal.

Pastes and Purees

Pastes and purees can be made from vegetable, but the most common types are tomato and garlic pastes, which are used in cooking. They are made by mashing any vegetable to a smooth, thick consistency and then carefully boiling this puree to evaporate the water with constant stirring to prevent burning. The concentration of solids in the final product is normally around 36%. This high solids content and the natural acidity preserve the product for several days, but they should be pasteurized for a longer shelf life. An alternative method for producing tomato paste is to hang the pulp in a sterilized cotton sack for an hour. The watery juice drains out and the pulp loses up to half its weight. 2.5% salt is mixed into the concentrate and it is re-hung for a further hour, during which time the weight falls to one-third of the original. The product can then be packaged and pasteurized or further concentrated by heating. This product has a more natural flavor and uses much less fuel than boiling.

Packaging

Traditional packaging materials such as baskets, jute sacks, and wooden boxes have long been established for packaging dried foods such as vegetables. Packaging is done for commodities which are transported in large quantities to a central marketing place and then sold loose. These packages can be used several times and are usually cheap.

Traditional packaging is only suitable provided the climate does not cause an increase in the moisture content of the food which will result in mould growth. If the climate is not suitable, dried foods should not be transported in this way. Boxes are used to prevent crushing of dried foods, and in humid climates, moisture-proof flexible films can be used.

Some semi-moist foods such as osmotically dried vegetables have special needs to prevent the reabsorption of water. Since dried fruit is a valuable product, it may be worth spending more on the package, such as a moisture-proof sealed bag. A wide range of flexible packaging materials is also available, but the use of many of these is limited due to high costs. Low-density polyethylene is a moderately good moisture barrier and cheaper than other films. It can be easily sealed using a powered bar-sealer.

Flexible materials may be used as the sole component of a package, but for most foods, a sturdy outer container is also needed to prevent crushing or to exclude light.

Flavor Compounds in Vegetables

The natural flavors of vegetables are due to presence of aldehydes, alcohol, ketones, organic acids and sulfur compounds. Some fruits and vegetables have an astringent taste attributed to phenolic compounds or tannins. Two types of vegetables, viz. vegetables belonging to the Allium and Cruciferae families have strong flavors resulting from the presence of various sulfur containing compounds.

Allium is the genus that includes onions and garlic. Vegetables belonging to the family Cruciferae, which include broccoli, cabbage, turnips and cauliflower, also contain prominent sulfur compounds. They are described as strong flavored vegetables. Vegetables of the onion family are usually strong flavored in the raw state and tend to lose some of the strong flavors when cooked in water.

Onions contain sulfur compounds that are acted upon by enzymes in the tissues when the vegetable is peeled or cut to eventually produce the volatile sulfur compounds that irritate the eyes and give biting and burning sensations on the tongue.

Vegetables of the cabbage family (cauliflower, cabbage, knolkhol) are relatively mild when raw but develop strong flavors when overcooked or improperly cooked. An amino acid S-methyl l-cysteine sulphoxide is also present in raw cabbage and appears to be a precursor of cooked cabbage flavor.

CONSERVATION OF NUTRIENTS IN PREPARATION AND COOKING OF VEGETABLES

Loss of nutrients in vegetables begins from preparation onward and is greater during the cooking process.

1. When vegetables are peeled the vitamins present under the skin may be lost.

2. Nutrients are also lost when the edible leaves of carrot beetroot and outer layer of cabbage are discarded.

3. Vitamin B complex and vitamin C are water soluble and are lost when the water in which vegetables are cooked is discarded. Sodium, potassium and chlorine are also lost when cooking water is discarded.

4. Vitamin C is lost by oxidation due to exposure of air.

5. During dehydration ascorbic acid and carotene are lost.

6. Addition of soda results in heavy loss of B vitamins during cooking.

Technology of Fruit Products

FRUITS

Fruit: Mature ovary of a flower.

The fleshy portion of the pericarp makes up the chief edible portion of the fruit.

Fruits can be classified as follows:

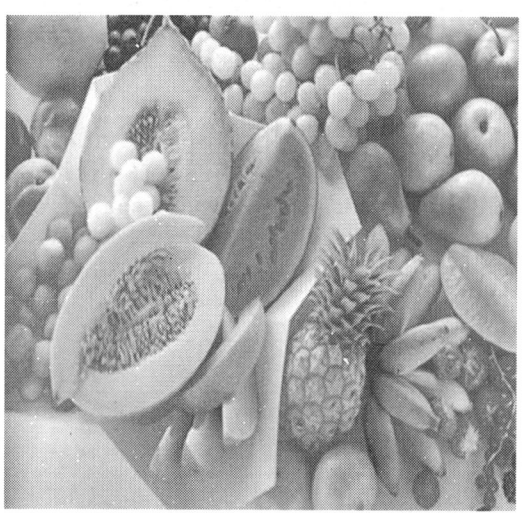

Simple Fruits

Containing one or more carpels, simple fruits, take roots from a single ovary and may or may not take in further modified accessory floral (perianth) structures. It will be either fleshy or dry; fleshy fruits include the berry, drupe and pome.

Compound Fruits

Fruits which are composed of two or more similar parts. They are also known as aggregate fruits.

Accessory Fruits

Accessory fruits are also called false fruit, spurious fruit, pseudo fruit, or pseudo carp.

Fruits are also classified as:

Citrus: Lemon, lime, orange, sweet lime.

Berries: Gooseberry, grapes, strawberry.

Drupes: Peach, plums, apricot.

Melons: Water melon, musk melon

Pomes: Apple, pear.

Berries

Berries are fruits with layers of pericarp (fruit coat), which are often homogenous, except for the skin on the outside. The pericarp layers are pulpous and juicy, and contain seeds embedded in the pulp mass. The fruits have fragile cell structure that is damaged by rough handling or freezing.

Citrus Fruits

These fruits belong to the genus *Citrus* which contains about 16 species of evergreen aromatic shrubs and trees mostly with thorny branches distributed throughout the tropical and subtropical regions of the world.

The common citrus fruits are orange, lemon and lime. The bright color, pleasing flavor and sweetness make them a favorite fruit. They are served as juice and can be eaten raw.

Drupes

Drupes are edible fruits with a thin skin, and juicy flesh enclosing a single seed (stone). Apricots, cherries, peaches and plums belong to this group.

Melons

Melons belong to the same family as cucumbers (Cucurbitaceae). Melons are commonly eaten raw. Their flesh consists of about 94% water and only 5% sugars. The seeds stripped of their hard coats may be eaten and also yield an edible oil.

Pomes

Pomes are fruits of apple and pear trees. The receptacle, surrounds the ovaries in the flower, enlarges to become edible and juicy, and encloses the cells containing the seeds. Fruits particularly citrus varieties and guava are a good source of vitamin C. Yellow fruits like mango and papaya contain β-carotene. Banana is a good source of carbohydrate and hence energy. Fruits are a poor source of protein and fat with the exception of avocado. Fruits also contain fiber and minerals such as sodium, potassium and magnesium. They are not a good source of calcium. Dry fruits, seethaphal and watermelon contribute appreciable amounts of iron.

PIGMENTS AND FLAVOR COMPOUNDS

Chlorophyll

The pigment responsible for green color of leafy vegetables and other green colored vegetables.

Carotenoids

The pigments responsible for yellow, orange, fat soluble pigments distributed in nature. They are divided into three groups, viz. carotenes present in carrot, green leafy vegetables and other fruits, lycopenes present in tomatoes and xanthophylls present in yellow fruits. Pigments that contain the phenolic group include anthocyanin, anthoxanthin, leucoanthoxanthin, catechin, quinones and betalins. The first four groups are collectively known as "Flavanoids".

Anthocyanin

They are water-soluble pigments responsible for red color occurring in many fruits. Apples, cherries, pomegranates have their color appeal due to anthocyanins.

Anthoxanthins

They are colorless white to yellow pigments that give color to cauliflower, onions, spinach or other leafy vegetables.

Leucoanthoxanthins

They are colorless and contribute to the puckeriness or astringency of some foods, such as apple and olives. They also play an important role in the enzymatic browning of fruits.

Catechins

They are pigments that are involved in enzymatic browning.

Betalins

They are the red water soluble pigments found in beetroot and berries.

Quinone

The yellow pigment juglone is a quinone present in walnut.

Mangiferin

This is the yellow pigment belonging to the xanthone group. It is found in mangoes.

Tannins

They are complex mixtures of polymeric polyphenols. The appearance of tannins ranges from colorless to yellow or brown. Tannins contribute to the astringency of foods and also to enzymatic browning.

Flavor Compounds

The flavor of fruits and vegetables are extremely important to their acceptance in the diet. The overall flavor impression is the result of the tastes perceived by the taste buds in the mouth and the aromatic compounds detected by the epithelium in the olfactory organ in the nose.

In fruits, sugars, acids, salts and bitter quinine-like compounds are tasted while the food is chewed in the mouth. Sweetness may result from the presence of glucose, galactose, fructose, ribose, arabinose and xylose. All fruits and vegetables contain a small amount of salt, which is detected in the overall taste impressions contributing to flavor.

PECTIN—ROLE IN GEL FORMATION

Pectin is the term designated to those water-soluble pectinic acids of varying methyl ester content. They are present in between cell walls in soft tissues of most plants acting as cementing substances.

In general it is the pulp and not the juice of fruits that contain pectin. Apples contain abundant pectin in their cores and skin. In the preparation of jams, the cores and skins are cooked with the pulp for pectin extraction. In citrus fruits, the pectin is chiefly in the white part of the rind. Other sources are sunflower seeds, guava and peels of mango and orange.

Heat is essential to extract the pectin. The usual way to extract the pectin from fruit is to heat the fruit in a small amount of water. Apples are cut into small pieces or ground with skin or core left intact and cooked to extract the maximum amount of pectin. Guavas are sliced thin and cooked with water to extract pectin.

Some Points to be Remembered for Extracting Pectin

- The maximum quantity of pectin is extracted in an acid solute. If fruits are rich in pectin but low in acidity, acidifying the solution before cooking increases the viscosity of the extraction.
- Cooked extractions contain more pectin than raw juices.
- Short periods of cooking (usually 10–20 minutes) results in formation of better jelly than does long boiling.

The Role of Pectin in Gel Formation

The formation of a firm jelly takes place only when pectin, acid and sugar and water are in definite proportions.

When sugar is added to the pectin solution, it acts as a dehydrating agent and destabilizes the pectin-water equilibrium and the pectin conglomerates forming a network of insoluble fibers. Large amounts of sugar solution can be held in this mesh-like structure.

The strength of the jelly depends on the structure of fibers, their continuity and rigidity. The continuity of the network depends upon the amount of pectin present in the system and the firmness depends on sugar concentration and acidity.

A soft jelly can be obtained by decreasing the amount of sugar. However, the rate of setting is modified by acidity. The fibrils of pectin become tough in the presence of an acid and thus able to hold the sugar solution in the interfibrillar spaces. If the amount of acid is large, the fibrils lose their elasticity and as a result jelly becomes syrupy.

Role of Fruits in Diet

1. Fruits provide vitamins and minerals required for growth and maintenance of health and are thus termed as protective foods.
2. Fruits provide nutrients and add variety to the diet. They make the diet attractive by their texture, flavor and color.
3. Fruits contain phytochemicals. The term phytochemicals refers to the wide variety of plant compounds naturally produced by plants. They include flavoring substances. Fruits with bright colors, viz. yellow, orange, red, green, blue, purple contain phytochemicals. Beta-carotene, vitamin C and vitamin E are nutrients that function as antioxidants. An antioxidant is a substance that significantly reduces or prevents oxidation of fatty acids and protein thus preventing cell and tissue damage caused by free radicals in the body.
4. Intake of fibrous fruits and vegetables are important as they:
   - Give satiety and thereby decrease food intake.
   - Help in regulating bowel movement.
   - Low in calorie content.
   - Reduce blood cholesterol levels.
   - Promote chewing and decrease rate of ingestion.
5. Fruits are used in the preparation of salads.

Fruit salad is a colorful, refreshing and light dessert. Pineapple, orange segments, apple cubes, papaya cubes, grapes, bananas, sapotas, mangoes, pomegranates are some of the fruits which can be used in a salad.

BROWNING

When fruits such as apple, banana, potato and brinjal are cut, there is a development of brown color on the surface due to action of enzymes. This is known as enzymatic browning. When the tissue is injured or cut and the cut surface is exposed to air, phenol oxidise enzymes are released at the surface.

These act with the polyphenols present in the fruits and oxidizes them to orthoquinones, which gives the brown color to cut tissues.

Browning can be prevented by the following methods:

1. Inactivation of polyphenol oxidise by applying heat.
2. Elimination of oxygen by vacuum packing.
3. Change of pH to prevent enzyme action.
4. Dipping of fruits and vegetables in brine and sugar solutions.
5. Use of antioxidants such as ascorbic acid to retard oxidation.

FRUIT PRODUCTS

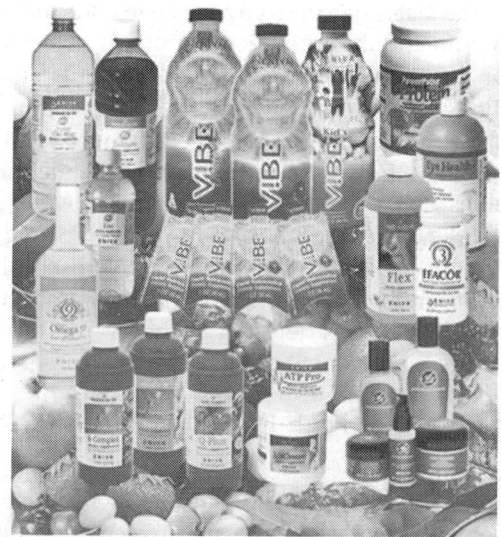

Jam

Jams are prepared by boiling fruit pulp with sufficient amount of sugar to a reasonably thick consistency, firm enough to hold the fruit tissue in position. Jam is made using pulp from a single fruit or from a mixture of fruits. The combination of high acidity (pH around 3.0) and high sugar content (68–72%), prevents mould growth after opening the jar.

In preparing jam, the fruit is crushed or finely cut and measured quantity of sugar and preservatives are added so that when cooked, the mass is fairly uniform throughout. Jams can be prepared from all varieties of pulpy fruits such as grapes, mango, sapota, banana, guava, etc. Jams should be hot filled (at around 85°C) into glass jars and sealed with a new lid. If the temperature is too high, steam condenses to water on the inside of the lid and dilutes sugar at the surface of the jam, which can cause mould growth. If the temperature is too low, the jam thickens and is difficult to pour into containers. Jars should be filled to approximately 9/10th full, to help a vacuum to form in the space above the product as it cools. The jars are kept upright during cooling until the gel has formed.

Jelly

The semisolid product prepared from boiling of clear solution of pectin containing fruit extract with addition of sugar and acid is jelly. Jellies are prepared by boiling fruits in water. The extract obtained is strained and measured quantity of sugar is added to it. The mixture is then boiled to a stage at which it will set to a clear gel.

Qualities of Good Jelly

- Transparent
- Well set
- Stiff
- Original flavor of the fruit.
- Retain its shape when removed from the mould.

Usually fruits such as guava, pineapple, apple, grape and a mixture of fruits rich in pectin can be used for the preparation of jellies.

Fruit Juices

Juice can be extracted from fruits in a number of ways, depending on the hardness of the raw material. Soft fruits such as berries can be pressed in a fruit press, or pulped using a juicer attachment to a food processor. Stea-

mers, such as those used for blanching, can also be used to 'dissolve' some types of cut soft fruits such as melon and pawpaw. Fruits can be heated in a wire basket in boiling water for 10 minutes to loosen the skin before pulping. Citrus fruits are usually reamed to extract the juice without the bitter pith or skin. Harder fruits, such as pineapple, are peeled and pulped using a liquidizer and pressed to extract the juice. Other fruit juices can be prepared using a pulper finisher that separates skins and seeds from the pulp. Seed bearing fruit should not be liquidized unless the seeds are removed first, because the fast-moving blades chop the seeds into small pieces that then appear to be contaminants. When a clearer juice is required it is necessary to filter it through a fine cloth or stainless steel juice strainer. A crystal clear juice requires a filter press, which is a considerable investment for a small-scale processor. Fruit beverages are prepared from different fruits such as apple, mango, grapes, lime, pineapple, sapota and in different forms such as pure juices, crushes, squashes and cordials.

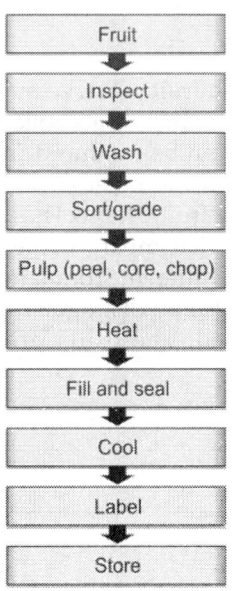

Process of preparing juice

The ratios of sugar and fruit juice in the preparation of various beverages are as follows:

Crushes: 25% fruit juice and 55% sugar.

Squashes: 25% fruit juice and 45% sugar.

Cordial: Clarified juice 1 liter and 250 gm sugar.

In the preparation of fruit juices, citric acid is usually added to clarify the sugar syrup. Preservatives such as sodium benzoate are added to tomato and grape juices while potassium metabisulphite (KMS) is added to all other fruit beverages.

Chutney

Chutneys are prepared by boiling sour fruits with sugar, spices and sometimes vinegar if there is a little acid in the fruit. If a dark product is required, sugar is added before heating, or it is added towards the end of boiling for a lighter product. The high sugar content and acid preserves the chutney after a jar has been opened. Some spices also have a preservative effect, in addition to contributing to the flavor of the chutney.

Marmalade

Marmalade is a fruit preserve made from the juice and peel of citrus fruits boiled with sugar and water. It can be produced from lemons, grapes, oranges and other citrus fruits or by mixing another fruit. The peel has a distinctive bitter taste which it imparts to the marmalade. Marmalade is different from jam by its fruit peel. It may also be distinguished from jam and fruits used. The fruits product order

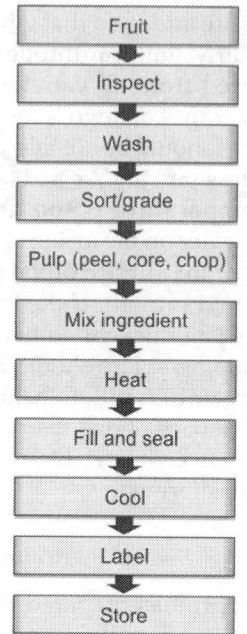

Process of making chutney

specifications for marmalade are TSS (65%) and fruit juice (45%) of the prepared product.

Ingredients: Pectin extract: 1 L

Sugar: 750 gm

Shredded peel: 62 gm

Qualities of Good Jelly

- Transparent
- Well set
- Stiff
- Good and original flavor
- Keep the shape when removed from mould.
- Sticky

Objective Questions

1500 One Word Objective Questions with Answers

▌ONE WORD QUESTIONS

1. What does the word "Nutrition" means?

    A. Swallowing food

    B. Eating food

    C. Ingestion and assimilation of nutrients

    D. Buying food

2. What is mean by the term "Food Safety?"

    A. Eating food in a safe manner

    B. Keeping food safe in the cupboard

    C. Eating vegetarian food

    D. Making sure the food you eat is safe and hygienic

3. Which one of these statements about bacteria is true?

    A. All types of bacteria give food poisoning

    B. Freezing makes food last longer by killing bacteria

    C. Bacteria grow fastest when they are warm

    D. All bacteria need air to survive

4. The temperature inside your fridge should be:

    A. 10°C

    B. 4°C

    C. 0°C

    D. –2°C

5. Which one of these foods is likely to contain the most bacteria?

    A. Cooked chicken

    B. Tinned cream

    C. Frozen raw chicken

    D. Bottled mayonnaise

6. Food poisoning bacteria will multiply readily between:

    A. –18°–0°C   B. 0°–5°C

    C. 5°–63°C   D. 63°–90°C

7. The temperature in your freezer should be:

    A. –2°C   B. –9°C

    C. –12°C   D. –18°C

8. At work, the best way to dry your hands after washing is:

    A. Using a warm air dryer

    B. Give them a shake

    C. Using a cotton towel

    D. Using a paper towel

9. Which of the following foods is a good source of fiber?

    A. A piece of pie

    B. Scrambled eggs

    C. Potato skin

    D. A cup of yogurt

10. Which of the following foods contains unsaturated fat?

   A. Cheese   B. Butter

   C. Steak   D. Olive oil

11. _____ is produced by fermentation involving lactic acid bacteria.

   A. Icecream

   B. Coffee

   C. Pudding

   D. Vinegar

12. What is the primary reason for blanching foods?

   A. Cleans the food

   B. Inactivates enzymes found in food

   C. Prevents pest infestation

   D. Prevents food from drying out

13. What is the operating principle behind oven drying for determining moisture content of foods?

   A. Color change is measured

   B. Loss of weight represents loss of water

   C. Change in refractive index is measured

   D. Change in light absorbance is measured

14. Which of the following packages is an example of aseptic packaging?

   A. Tetra Pak drinking boxes

   B. Paper bag

   C. Milk carton

   D. Plastic bread bag

15. Which gas causes fruits to ripen?

   A. Carbon monoxide

   B. Nitrogen

   C. Propane

   D. Ethylene

16. Which of the following does not affect the basal metabolism rate of a human being is?

   A. Diet   B. Size

   C. Sex   D. Age

17. A calorie is the amount of energy required to raise _____ of water one degree _____.

   A. 1 ounce, fahrenheit

   B. 1 gram, centigrade

   C. 1 kilo, fahrenheit

   D. 1 gram, centigrade

18. Carbohydrates supply _____ kcal per gram.

   A. 4   B. 5

   C. 6   D. 7

19. Which is not preserved by bacteria?

   A. Yogurt   B. Bread

   C. Wine   D. Whole milk

20. Bacteria can grow in an all except _____.

   A. Sugar   B. Milk

   C. Meat   D. Vegetables

21. What is used by technologists to make some ready-to-eat cereals_____?

   A. Flaking and shredding

   B. Inflaking and inshredding

   C. Posting and kellogging

   D. Extending and fluffing

22. Fatty acid does not contain which of the following elements?

   A. Oxygen

   B. Carbon

   C. Nitrogen

   D. Hydrogen

23. In which of the following foods solanine (toxin) is present?

   A. Tomato   B. Coffee

   C. Potato   D. Tea

24. The main function of an emulsifier _____.

   A. Prevents the separation of oil and water in food

   B. Maintains the shape or crispness of fruits and vegetables

   C. Controls insects and pests

   D. Produces or stimulates CO_2 production

25. _____ is a food additive that retards rancidity of unsaturated oils and prevents browning in fruits and vegetables that occur during exposure to oxygen.

A. Anti-caking free-flowing agent

B. Antimicrobial agent

C. Antioxidant

D. Anti-buffer agent

26. A system that is used to enhance food safety in food processing, packaging, storage, distribution, and preparation is _____.

A. Good manufacturing practices

B. Hazard analysis and critical control point

C. High accuracy and contamination control point

D. Best management practices

27. _____ are places in the food processing system where the lack of proper control can result in a safety risk for the consumer.

A. Concentrated contamination control processes

B. Critical control points

C. Critical contamination places

D. Contamination processing points

28. A bacteria that can contaminate poultry products and cause food borne illness in humans is_____.

A. Lactobacillus

B. Clostridium

C. Salmonella

D. Gram-positive

29. _____ is the most effective way to eliminate living microorganisms in spices.

A. Freezing

B. Heat

C. Irradiation

D. Selected chemicals

30. An addition of a nutrient to foods such as adding vitamin A to milk is called _____.

A. Irradiation   B. Nitrification

C. Fortification   D. Fermentation

31. Main factors responsible for rancidity are _____.

A. Freezing

B. Irradiation

C. Heat

D. Selected chemicals

32. Lactic acid bacteria can ferment sugars and nutrients in pickles because _____.

A. Use a natural occurring enzyme

B. Produce lactic acid

C. Are tolerant of salt levels

D. Use acetic acid

33. Food label is mentioned with a list of food ingredients. The first ingredient listed is by its amount of:

A. Percent protein

B. Grams of carbohydrates

C. Total weight

D. Fat content

34. _____ helps in production of soy sauce.

A. Mold   B. Bacteria

C. Fungi   D. Yeast

35. Fats and oils are part of a family of compounds called _____.

A. Proteins   B. Carbohydrates

C. Lipids   D. Fiber

36. Measurement of relative number of hydrogen and hydroxide ions in a food system. This is also known as _____.

A. Water activity

B. Brix

C. Sodium concentration

D. pH

37. Change in the shape of a protein molecule without breaking its covalent bonds is called _____.
    A. Coagulation   B. Denaturation
    C. Agglutination   D. Saturation

38. _____ is the complete destruction of all microorganisms, except some bacterial spores.
    A. Pasteurization
    B. Commercial sterilization
    C. Irradiation
    D. Sterilization

39. A _____ is an illness caused by consuming a food that contains a harmful metabolite from a microorganism.
    A. Food borne intoxication
    B. Bacteriocide
    C. Bacteriostat
    D. Food borne infection

40. A synthetic sweetener made of aspartic acid and phenylalanine that is found in many diet soft drinks is called _____.
    A. Sorbitol   B. Asparatame
    C. Saccharin   D. Cyclamates

41. _____ is also known as baking soda.
    A. Carbon dioxide
    B. Potassium bitartrate
    C. Calcium carbonate
    D. Sodium bicarbonate

42. The use of biochemical techniques to alter the genetic makeup of a plant to enhance characteristics for food production is called _____.
    A. Biogenetics   B. Biotechnology
    C. Biophysiology   D. Biophysics

43. When fruits and vegetables are bruised or cut, discoloration occurs. This is called _____.
    A. Caramelization
    B. Sulfating

C. Dehydration
D. Enzymatic browning

44. 2 gm of fat, 6 gm of carbohydrates and 5 gm of protein will provide _____ calories.
    A. 62   B. 108
    C. 93   D. 113

45. Soft drinks prepared are added with Sodium benzoate. It inhibit the growth of _____.
    A. Rancidity
    B. Color deterioration
    C. Mold growth
    D. Flavor breakdown

46. The deficiency of vitamin D leads to _____.
    A. Scurvy   B. Rickets
    C. Pellagra   D. Beriberi

47. GMP stands for _____.
    A. Get more practice
    B. Good manufacturing procedures
    C. Good manufacturing practices
    D. Good methods procedures

48. Leavening agents such as baking soda or baking powder in cakes and cookies are added to provide _____.
    A. Sodium dioxide
    B. Carbon dioxide
    C. Sodium monoxide
    D. Carbon monoxide

49. _____ is present in higher amounts in fruits and vegetables.
    A. Carbohydrates   B. Water
    C. Protein   D. Fat

50. As per the law _____ should be mentioned on all food labels.
    A. The product price
    B. Preparation instructions
    C. The quantity
    D. Suggested uses

51. _____ is the protein in meat, primarily responsible for meat color.

   A. Myosin   B. Actin
   C. Myoglobin   D. Hemoglobin

52. Technically freeze drying is known as _____.

   A. Sublimation
   B. Lyophilization
   C. Condensation
   D. Evaporation

53. The globular protein found in milk is _____.

   A. Casein   B. Keratin
   C. Elastin   D. Gluten

54. _____ is elastic, stretchy protein found in wheat.

   A. Casein   B. Avidin
   C. Gluten   D. Albumin

55. Processed food products such as cereals and orange juice may be fortified to enhance their nutritional content:

   A. Stabilizers
   B. Chelators
   C. Vitamins and minerals
   D. Antioxidants

56. When fruits such as apples or bananas are cut, the cut surface becomes brown. This is due to _____.

   A. The Maillard reaction
   B. Enzymatic browning
   C. Exposure to light
   D. Catabolism

57. An _____ can be used to keep water and oil mixed together in solution.

   A. Invertase   B. Caking agent
   C. Emulsifier   D. Antimicrobial

58. HTST is a method of pasteurization of milk. HTST is _____.

   A. Homogenous tempering short time
   B. High temperature short time

C. Hot temperature short tempering
D. Homogenization time speeding temperature

59. For curing meat _____ is added which serve as an antibotulinal agent.

   A. Sodium erythorbate
   B. Sodium benzoate
   C. Sodium nitrite
   D. Sodium chloride

60. To determine the amount of free water available for microbes to use in a food system, a food scientist would measure the _____ of that food.

   A. Water activity   B. Percent water
   C. pH   D. Brix

61. To measure the texture of a wheat dough, a food technologist might use a:

   A. Apiral plater
   B. Gas chromatograph
   C. Blender
   D. Texture analyzer

62. _____ is responsible for the red color of a tomato.

   A. Beta carotene   B. Lycopene
   C. Limonene   D. Myosin

63. _____ are the building blocks of proteins.

   A. Amino acids   B. Monosaccharides
   C. Fatty acids   D. Lipids

64. Coagulation of milk occurs in the presence of enzyme _____.

   A. Rennet   B. Amylase
   C. Trypsin   D. Cysteine

65. The meat of swine is known as _____.

   A. Pork   B. Mutton
   C. Chicken   D. Beaf

66. Papaya contains the enzyme _____.

   A. Pepsin   B. Papain
   C. Peptidase   D. Proteolase

67. _____ is a enzyme present in pineapple.
 A. Phosphatase   B. Papain
 C. Bromelain   D. Pepsin

68. Darkening of tamarind pulp is due to _____.
 A. Denaturation of proteins
 B. Oxidation of carbohydrates
 C. Breakdown of fatty acids
 D. Oxidation of phenolic compounds

69. The fermentation of milk occurs in the presence of _____ bacteria.
 A. Salmonella
 B. Lactobacillus
 C. Streptococcus
 D. *Clostridium botulinum*

70. The rearing and management of fishes on large scale is called _____.
 A. Vermiculture
 B. Pisciculture
 C. Epiculture
 D. Composting

71. Cheese curd is primarily composed of coagulated:
 A. Lactose   B. Protein
 C. Fat   D. Carbohydrate

72. Chemically table salt is known as _____.
 A. Sodium bicarbonate
 B. Potassium nitrate
 C. Sodium bisulfite
 D. Sodium chloride

73. _____ is not the function of antioxidants.
 A. Color preservation
 B. Preventing protein degradation
 C. Minimizing rancidity
 D. Preserving flavor

74. Corn and peanuts contains the _____ toxin.
 A. Solanine   B. Protease
 C. Aflatoxins   D. Cyanide

75. Red meat and poultry are good sources of _____.
 A. Ash   B. Calcium
 C. Protein   D. Carbohydrates

76. The ingredient _____ is added to impart a unique color and flavor to cured meat products.
 A. Sodium chloride
 B. Sodium nitrate
 C. Sodium citrate
 D. Sodium nitrite

77. It combines with the iron to produce hemoglobin in the body:
 A. Copper   B. Zinc
 C. Sulphur   D. Sodium

78. Which of the bacteria can grow in alkaline pH?
 A. Lactobacilli   B. *Vibrio cholerae*
 C. Salmonella   D. Staphylococcus

79. The percentage fat constituent of double toned milk is:
 A. 0.5   B. 1.5
 C. 3.0   D. 4.5

80. Which of the following microorganisms is commonly known as 'Pink Bread Mould'?
 A. Neurospora   B. Aspergillus
 C. Mucor   D. Rhizopus

81. If a product is said to be "Sugar free" it contains how much sugar?
 A. None
 B. Less than 0.5 gm of sugar per serving
 C. Less than 10.0 gm
 D. Not more than 40 kcal per serving

82. Vitamin C and vitamin E, BHA and BHT, and sulfites are all:
 A. Falvor enhancer
 B. Antimicrobial agent
 C. Incidental food agent
 D. Antioxidants

83. For the first time, bacteria were observed by:
   A. WH Stanley
   B. Louis Pasteur
   C. Robert Koch
   D. AV Leewenhoek

84. Smallest unit of proteins is:
   A. Fatty acid   B. Amino acid
   C. Glycogen   D. All of the above

85. The enzymes present in gastric juice:
   A. Pepsin   B. Trypsin
   C. Lipase   D. All of the above

86. Vitamin B is necessary for preventing:
   A. Beriberi   B. Night blindness
   C. Scurvy   D. Goiter

87. World Health Organization was established on:
   A. 1945   B. 1948
   C. 1955   D. 1958

88. Balanced diet is:
   A. Easily digestible
   B. Nutritionally adequate
   C. Healthy
   D. All of the above

89. The vitamin necessary for eyes is:
   A. Vitamin A   B. Vitamin B
   C. Vitamin C   D. Vitamin D

90. The component of diet necessary for the growth of the body:
   A. Carbohydrate   B. Protein
   C. Vitamin   D. Minerals

91. For preventing goiter, _____ is necessary in diet.
   A. Iodine   B. Phosphorus
   C. Vitamin C   D. Proteins

92. Citrus fruits are good sources of
   A. Vitamin C   B. Vitamin D
   C. Vitamin A   D. Vitamin E

93. The electrolyte balance is maintained in body through:
   A. Proteins   B. Water
   C. Vitamins   D. Fiber

94. The diet deficient in all the nutrients will lead to:
   A. Malnutrition   B. Undernutrition
   C. Good nutrition   D. A and B both

95. The deficiency of iron leads to:
   A. Lack of blood
   B. Growth retardation
   C. Weakness
   D. All of the above

96. Wrong cooking practices results in:
   A. Loss of nutrients B. Nutritious food
   C. Good health   D. All of the above

97. Goiter is caused by deficiency of:
   A. Excess of iodine
   B. Deficiency of iodine
   C. Lack of vitamin A
   D. All of the above

98. Deficiency of vitamin B_1 leads to:
   A. Beriberi   B. Night blindness
   C. Scurvy   D. Rickets

99. Deficiency of vitamin C leads to:
   A. Pellagra   B. Rickets
   C. Scurvy   D. Edema

100. Enzyme present in saliva:
   A. Salivary amylase
   B. Lipase
   C. Protease
   D. Pepsin

101. The proteins present in wheat is:
   A. Niacin   B. Threonine
   C. Gluten   D. Methionine

102. Lactose is found in:
   A. Milk   B. Pulses
   C. Vegetables   D. Fruits

103. Kwashiorkor is caused due to deficiency of:

    A. Proteins

    B. Carbohydrates

    C. Vitamin D

    D. All of the above

104. Deficiency of fats leads to:

    A. Obesity   B. Phrynoderma

    C. Anemia   D. Osteoporosis

105. 1 gm of fats gives _____ calories.

    A. 4 kcal   B. 5 kcal

    C. 9 kcal   D. 10 kcal

106. Deficiency of vitamin D leads to:

    A. Night blindness

    B. Rickets

    C. Goiter

    D. Anemia

107. The function of food is:

    A. Provide energy to the body

    B. Growth of body

    C. Prevention from diseases

    D. All of the above

108. Amla is a very good source of:

    A. Vitamin C

    B. Vitamin A

    C. Vitamin D

    D. Vitamin K

109. _____ is the protein present in rice.

    A. Albumin   B. Gluten

    C. Arginine   D. Globulin

110. The protein present in corn is called _____.

    A. Arginine   B. Zein

    C. Glydine   D. Collagen

111. Chemical components present in diet, which performs various functions in body:

    A. Nutrients   B. Food groups

    C. Fiber   D. None of the above

112. The term food means:

    A. Which nourishes the body

    B. Removes hunger

    C. Gives satisfaction

    D. All of the above

113. The desirable weight of the individual depends on:

    A. Bone structure

    B. Body fat content

    C. Muscular development

    D. All of the above

114. Vitamin D deficiency leads to:

    A. Osteomalacia

    B. Rickets

    C. Osteoporosis

    D. All of the above

115. The _____ pigment is responsible for yellow color of fruits and vegetables.

    A. Litmus   B. Chlorophyll

    C. Carotene   D. None of the above

116. The conversion of carotene into vitamin A takes place in:

    A. Intestine   B. Liver

    C. Gallbladder   D. Stomach

117. _____ is an infection of the ligaments and bones that support the teeth. This causes red gums, or bleeding when you brush or floss.

    A. Cirrhosis   B. Rickets

    C. Pyorrhea   D. Diarrhea

118. The vitamin that is made in the body by the action of sunrays on the fat under the skin:

    A. Vitamin D   B. Vitamin C

    C. Vitamin A   D. Vitamin B

119. The mineral which combines with iron to produce hemoglobin in the body:

    A. Copper   B. Zinc

    C. Sulphur   D. Sodium

120. _____ cereal is rich in vitamin A.
  A. Yellow maize   B. Bajra
  C. Rice   D. Wheat

121. Parboiled rice contains good amount of _____.
  A. Niacin   B. Thiamine
  C. Ascorbic acid   D. All of the above

122. The people who eat mostly corn often suffers from:
  A. Kwashiorkor   B. Rickets
  C. Pellagra   D. Night blindness

123. _____ is present in tomato.
  A. Chlorophyll   B. Lycopene
  C. Xanthophyll   D. All of the above

124. Fresh citrus fruits are good sources of _____.
  A. Vitamin A   B. Vitamin C
  C. Vitamin K   D. Vitamin B

125. Papaya and mango are good sources of _____.
  A. Vitamin B   B. Vitamin A
  C. Vitamin C   D. Vitamin D

126. _____ is the structural and functional unit of life.
  A. Cell   B. Mitochondria
  C. Tissue   D. Organ

127. _____ is defined as the synthesis of compounds needed for use in the body.
  A. Photosynthesis B. Utilization
  C. Nutrition   D. Anabolism

128. _____ is defined as the breakdown of complex substances to simpler ones.
  A. Anabolism   B. Catabolism
  C. Obesity   D. Malnutrition

129. Breaking up of food in the intestinal tract is:
  A. Hydrolysis   B. Synthesis
  C. Digestion   D. Excretion

130. _____ is the process which carries the nutrients into the circulating system and delivers into the system.
  A. Assimilation   B. Absorption
  C. Digestion   D. Secretion

131. Digestion of proteins starts in:
  A. Intestine   B. Mouth
  C. Stomach   D. Liver

132. Milk is clotted by special enzyme called:
  A. Pepsin   B. Rennin
  C. Sucrose   D. Maltose

133. Starch is partly hydrolyzed by enzyme in the mouth:
  A. Salivary amylase (ptyalin)
  B. Pepsin
  C. Rennin
  D. Lipase

134. Hyperlipidemia is:
  A. Elevated level of blood fats
  B. Elevated level of blood proteins
  C. Elevated level of blood urea
  D. Elevated level of blood sugar

135. The process through which unsaturated acids are converted into saturated fats:
  A. Hydrolysis
  B. Hydrogenation
  C. Catalysis
  D. All of the above

136. Consumption of khesari dal leads to disease:
  A. Pellagra   B. Anemia
  C. Beriberi   D. Lathyrism

137. The energy released in the body from food is measured as a unit:
  A. Gram   B. kcal
  C. Milligram   D. Celsius

138. The organ in which glycogen is stored:
  A. Liver   B. Stomach
  C. Pancreas   D. Spleen

139. _____ vitamin is responsible for enhancing immunity.

A. Vitamins A and C

B. Vitamins D and K

C. Vitamins E and B

D. All of the above

140. Chemically vitamin B_1 is called:

A. Riboflavin   B. Niacin

C. Calciferol   D. Thiamine

141. Ripening of fruits occur due to presence of:

A. Oxygen   B. Carbon dioxide

C. Ethylene gas   D. Mono-oxide

142. _____ pigment is present in the beets and radish.

A. Anthocyanin   B. Flavones

C. Chlorophyll   D. Flavanol

143. Poultry foods are:

A. Chicken

B. Ducks and geese

C. Turkey and pigeons

D. All of the above

144. Rigor mortis is:

A. Physical activity

B. Cell chemical reaction

C. Stiffening of the carcass

D. None of the above

145. Puffed rice, wheat, popcorns, are examples of:

A. Wet cooking   B. Dry cooking

C. Gelatinization   D. None of the above

146. _____ is a process in which the change in color and physical state occurs when starch is heated in water.

A. Coagulation   B. Gel

C. Gelatinization   D. None of the above

147. The science which deals with the process of prevention of decay or spoilage of food

thus allowing it to be stored in a filth condition for future use:

A. Adulteration   B. Prevention

C. Poisoning   D. None of the above

148. Vitamin B_2 is also called:

A. Ascorbic acid   B. Phylloquinone

C. Riboflavin   D. Calciferol

149. Pyridoxine is:

A. Vitamin B_6 B. Vitamin C

C. Vitamin D   D. Vitamin E

150. Cyanocobalamin is:

A. Vitamin B_6 B. Vitamin B_{12}

C. Vitamin C   D. Vitamin D

151. For nourishment and disease free life diet is necessary:

A. Balanced diet

B. Low nutrient diet

C. High nutrient diet

D. Fat free diet

152. For growing child the diet should contain good quality rich foods:

A. Protein   B. Fat

C. Fiber   D. None of the above

153. Vitamin C is necessary for preventing:

A. Scurvy   B. Rickets

C. Osteomalacia   D. Beriberi

154. Vitamin is necessary for reproduction:

A. Vitamin B   B. Vitamin E

C. Vitamin A   D. Vitamin D

155. _____ is the energy giving component of food.

A. Minerals   B. Proteins

C. Vitamins   D. Carbohydrates

156. Term vitamin was coined by:

A. Mendel

B. M Swaminathan

C. Funk

D. Watson and Crick

157. PEM is:
    A. Protein energy measles
    B. Pulse energy malnutrition
    C. Protein energy malnutrition
    D. None of the above

158. The two major forms of PEM are:
    A. Kwashiorkor and marasmus
    B. Scurvy and pellagra
    C. Night blindness and xerosis
    D. All of the above

159. Anemia occurs due to deficiency of:
    A. Selenium   B. Molybdenum
    C. Iron   D. Sulfur

160. Gastric juice are secreted by stomach contains:
    A. Hydrochloric acid
    B. Pepsin
    C. Rennin
    D. All of the above

161. Fat soluble vitamins are:
    A. Vitamins A, D, E, and K
    B. Vitamins B, C
    C. Both
    D. None of the above

162. Water soluble vitamins are:
    A. Vitamin B   B. Vitamin C
    C. Both A and B   D. None of the above

163. Lipoproteins are synthesized in:
    A. Pancreas   B. Liver
    C. Stomach   D. Gallbladder

164. Low density lipoprotein (LDL) is:
    A. Bad cholesterol
    B. New cholesterol
    C. Good cholesterol
    D. None of the above

165. High density lipoprotein (HDL) is:
    A. Bad cholesterol
    B. Good cholesterol

C. Neutral cholesterol
D. None of the above

166. Basal metabolic rate is affected by:
    A. Age   B. Growth
    C. Sleep   D. All of the above

167. The study of science of nutrients deals with:
    A. What nutrients we need
    B. How much we need
    C. Why we need
    D. All of the above

168. Signs of good nutritional status are:
    A. An alert body with healthy skin
    B. Good natured personality, reddish pink color of cheeks
    C. Firm muscles
    D. All of the above

169. Pepsin, rennin and lipase are the enzymes secreted by:
    A. Pancreas   B. Stomach
    C. Liver   D. Esophagus

170. Cellulose, hemicelluloses and lignin are the major forms are:
    A. Carbohydrates   B. Proteins
    C. Fats   D. Vitamins

171. Casein, albumin and gluten are examples of:
    A. Carbohydrates   B. Proteins
    C. Fats   D. Minerals

172. Pellagra is caused by the deficiency of:
    A. Niacin   B. Thiamine
    C. Iron   D. Calcium

173. During school age the nutrients required are:
    A. Proteins   B. Minerals
    C. Vitamins   D. All of the above

174. For infant mother's milk is:
    A. Easily digestible and nutritious
    B. Indigestible

C. Hard

D. None of the above

175. Mother's milk contains _____ which prevents diseases and infections in infant.

A. Vitamins   B. Antibodies

C. Calcium   D. Magnesium

176. The stage when the mother breastfeed her infant is called:

A. Pregnancy

B. Lactating phase

C. Both A and B

D. None of the above

177. The first milk secreted from the breast of mother's milk after the infant is born, is called:

A. Prolactin   B. Colostrum

C. Cortisone   D. Thyroxin

178. For prevention of adulteration government of India created standards which are:

A. AGMARK

B. ISI

C. Both of the above

D. None of the above

179. Full form of AGMARK is:

A. Agricultural marketing

B. Agriculture market

C. Agro-marketing

D. None of the above

180. ISI is expanded as:

A. International Standard Institute

B. Indian Standard Institute

C. Both A and B

D. None of the above

181. _____ products are formed after digestion of proteins, which are absorbed by the tissues.

A. Amino acids   B. Carbohydrates

C. Vitamin A   D. Calcium

182. Aspartame and saccharin are the:

A. Fats

B. Artificial sweeteners

C. Both A and B

D. None of the above

183. One gram of fat gives how much calories:

A. 2 kcal   B. 8 kcal

C. 9 kcal   D. 4 kcal

184. Cereals, roots and fruits are _____ sources of vitamin (B_2).

A. Riboflavin   B. Very good

C. Good   D. Poor

185. Cheilosis and angular stomatitis are the symptoms of:

A. Vitamin C deficiency

B. Vitamin B_1 deficiency

C. Vitamin B_6 deficiency

D. Vitamin B_2 deficiency

186. Spongy and bleeding gums are the signs of:

A. Rickets   B. Night blindness

C. Scurvy   D. Beriberi

187. Important functions of minerals are:

A. Maintenance of acid–base balance

B. Control of water balance

C. Contraction of muscles

D. All of the above

188. Iron is stored in the liver, spleen and bone marrow in the form of:

A. Zinc   B. Carbohydrates

C. Cholesterol   D. Protein ferritin

189. Susceptibility to fractures of hip and wrist are the signs of:

A. Osteoporosis   B. Scurvy

C. Beriberi   D. Anemia

190. _____ plays an important role in the formation of antibodies.

A. Vitamin C   B. Vitamin D

C. Vitamin B_6 D. Vitamin E

191. The functions of water are:
    A. Universal solvent
    B. Maintaining electrolyte balance
    C. Transportation of nutrients to the cells
    D. All of the above

192. When intake of water and other fluids is less than the body intake _____ occurs.
    A. Dehydration
    B. Edema
    C. Rehydration
    D. None of the above

193. For the formation of red blood cells and hemoglobin _____ is important.
    A. Vitamins
    B. Proteins
    C. Carbohydrates
    D. Fats

194. The deficiency of proteins in small children leads to:
    A. Scurvy
    B. Beriberi
    C. Kwashiorkor
    D. Rickets

195. _____ are the good sources of vitamin A and vitamin D.
    A. Fish
    B. Egg
    C. Meat
    D. None of the above

196. Frequent urination is a sign of:
    A. Anemia
    B. Diabetes
    C. Glycosuria
    D. None of the above

197. Low protein diet during pregnancy leads to:
    A. Effect milk secretion
    B. Cause of anemia
    C. Nutritional edema
    D. All of the above

198. Important principles of diet therapy are:
    A. Knowledge about the patient
    B. Duration of illness
    C. Diet with variety based on likes and dislikes
    D. All of the above

199. Atherosclerosis caused by excessive intake of cholesterol makes:
    A. Heart enlarged
    B. Blood thick
    C. Blood vessels narrow and hardened
    D. None of the above

200. The nutritive value of cereals is effected by:
    A. Processing
    B. Milling
    C. Cooking
    D. All of the above

201. The green part of a sprouting potato contains a poison called:
    A. Alanine
    B. Solanine
    C. Iodine
    D. Aflatoxin

202. BMI is:
    A. Body multiple index
    B. Basal mass index
    C. Body mass index
    D. Basal measure index

203. The formula for calculating BMI is:
    A. Weight/height
    B. Weight (kg)/height $(m)^2$
    C. Weight/height^2
    D. Height/weight

203. An agency of India engaged in periodic diet and nutrition surveys is:
    A. Indian Council of Medical Research
    B. World Health Organization
    C. Food and Agricultural Organization
    D. National Nutrition Monitoring Bureau

204. World diabetes day falls on:
    A. 14th November
    B. 15th March
    C. 24th March
    D. 24th December

205. The specific odor of garlic is due to presence of:
    A. Chlorine containing compounds
    B. Fluorine containing compounds

C. Nitrogen-containing compounds

D. Sulfur-containing compounds

206. World consumer's right day falls on:

A. 15th March   B. 15th June

C. 26th October   D. 26th December

207. Complete food is:

A. Fruits   B. Vegetable

C. Milk   D. Pulses

208. The proteins found in bone is:

A. Collagen   B. Myosin

C. Hordein   D. Zein

209. The substance responsible for jelly making in fruits is:

A. Protein   B. Phytin

C. Pectin   D. Carotene

210. Foods are spoiled by the action of:

A. Microorganisms   B. Enzymes

C. Insects   D. All of the above

211. The scientific term for "cracking at the angles of the mouth":

A. Glossitis

B. Angular stomatitis

C. Dermatitis

D. Pellagra

212. Human milk is a poor source of:

A. Iron   B. Protein

C. Vitamin K   D. Vitamin B_{12}

213. Kwashiorkor and marasmus are associated with:

A. Insanitary condition

B. Total undernutrition

C. Protein-energy malnutrition

D. Vitamin C deficiency

214. The term IDD (iodine deficiency disorder) is introduced by:

A. Davis

B. Osborne and Mendel

C. Hetzel

D. Mulder

215. Normal blood glucose level of a healthy person is:

A. 60–90 mg/100 ml

B. 70–100 mg/100 ml

C. 80–120 mg/100 ml

D. 120–160 mg/100 ml

216. Insulin is useful for:

A. Reducing the weight

B. Lowering blood cholesterol

C. Lowering blood glucose level

D. Increase blood glucose level

217. Which of the following is a good source of cholesterol?

A. Spinach   B. Egg

C. Rice   D. Groundnut

218. Which of these food items provide empty calories?

A. Sugar   B. Potato

C. Egg   D. Groundnut

219. Which of the following is an example of dry heating method?

A. Broiling   B. Blanching

C. Stewing   D. Poaching

220. The red color of tomato is due to presence of:

A. Anthocyanin   B. Carotenoids

C. Lycopene   D. Chlorophyll

221. Full form of FPO is:

A. Food Products Order

B. Fruits Product Order

C. Fruit Preservation Order

D. Food Preservation Order

222. Which of the following compounds is added to the oil to avoid rancidity?

A. Vitamin A   B. BHT

C. BHA   D. Vitamin C

223. Candling is a method used to assess the quality of:
   A. Milk
   B. Meat
   C. Eggs
   D. Fish

224. Following is not a sensory quality characteristics:
   A. Appearance
   B. Color
   C. Seed weight
   D. Flavor

225. Snacks like chat and beverage are most suitable for serving in a:
   A. Hospital
   B. Old age home
   C. Orphanage
   D. College and school canteen

226. Food poisoning is an illness caused by:
   A. Microorganisms
   B. Toxins present in food
   C. Certain plants and animals
   D. None of the above

227. Amoebic dysentery is caused by:
   A. Bacteria
   B. Virus
   C. Protozoa
   D. Fungi

228. Following is a natural food:
   A. Sauce
   B. Pickle
   C. Wheat flour
   D. Apple

229. Characteristics of food which can be identified by use of our senses:
   A. Sensory evaluation
   B. Chemical qualities
   C. Physical qualities
   D. Palatability

230. Following proteins are present in egg yolk:
   A. Lipovitellins
   B. Phosvitin
   C. Livetin
   D. All of the above

231. Egg white contain _____ proteins.
   A. Ovalbumin
   B. Conalbumin
   C. Ovamucoid
   D. All of the above

232. The mineral which is required for the formation of bones and teeth is:
   A. Calcium
   B. Iron
   C. Vitamin A
   D. Selenium

233. Mushroom poisoning show symptoms of:
   A. Abdominal pain
   B. Nausea
   C. Vomiting and loose stools with blood
   D. All of the above

234. Which of the following nutrients is needed to build and maintain the structural components of the body?
   A. Carbohydrates
   B. Proteins
   C. Fat
   D. Fiber

235. Which of the following nutrients is known as the sunshine vitamin?
   A. Vitamin A
   B. Vitamin B
   C. Vitamin D
   D. Vitamin C

236. All of the following are needed for strong bones *except*:
   A. Thiamine
   B. Calcium
   C. Vitamin D
   D. Magnesium

237. This nutrient is needed for a healthy immune system:
   A. Fiber
   B. Vitamin K
   C. Fluoride
   D. Vitamin C

238. This mineral is essential for healthy red blood cells and a deficiency might cause anemia:
   A. Iron
   B. Magnesium
   C. Iodine
   D. Chromium

239. This vitamin is needed to prevent a birth defect called spina bifida:
   A. Vitamin A
   B. Calcium
   C. Folate
   D. Vitamin E

240. The vitamin is most important for healthy vision:
   A. Vitamin K
   B. Iron
   C. Calcium
   D. Vitamin A

241. The disease related to stomach is:
    A. Diverticulosis
    B. Flatulence
    C. Piles
    D. None of the above

242. The fiber should be included in:
    A. Piles   B. Flatulence
    C. Diverticulosis   D. None of the above

243. All except one are true about significance of dietary fiber:
    A. It promotes peristalsis
    B. Reduces cholesterol absorption
    C. Increases glycemic index
    D. Acts as an antioxidant

244. Human must easily tolerate a lack of which of the following nutrient?
    A. Proteins   B. Carbohydrates
    C. Fats   D. Fiber

245. Which of the nutrient is rich in medium- and short chain fatty acids?
    A. Milk   B. Peanut oil
    C. Sunflower oil   D. Almond oil

246. Which of the following is not a part of dietary fiber?
    A. Cellulose   B. Pectin
    C. Lignin   D. Agar

247. Which of the following has the highest specific dynamic action?
    A. Egg   B. Potato
    C. Corn oil   D. Mango

248. Which of the following has the highest glycemic index?
    A. Ice cream   B. Cucumber
    C. Bread   D. Dextrose

249. In a child suffering from marasmus, which of the following clinical manifestations is not observed:
    A. Watery diarrhea with acid stools
    B. Subnormal temperature
    C. Visible peristalsis from thin abdomibal wall
    D. Generalized edema

250. Blood pressure is related to which of the organ?
    A. Bones   B. Intestine
    C. Heart   D. Lungs

251. The vitamin which helps in clotting of blood?
    A. Vitamin A   B. Vitamin K
    C. Vitamin B   D. Vitamin D

252. The normal body temperature of human body is:
    A. 90.3°F   B. 98.4°F
    C. 100°F   D. 105°F

253. In fever the glycogen level in body:
    A. Reduces   B. Increases
    C. Remains stable   D. None of the above

254. For maintaining the level of glycogen in body, one must take enough:
    A. Vitamin A   B. Proteins
    C. Carbohydrates   D. Fats

255. In fever, metabolism of proteins:
    A. Increases
    B. Reduces
    C. Remains stable
    D. No and change occurs

256. Which disease occurs for short time with high fever?
    A. Pneumonia   B. Typhoid
    C. Malaria   D. Smallpox

257. In which disease balanced and nutritious diet is required?
    A. Pneumonia   B. Typhoid
    C. Malaria   D. Smallpox

258. Which devices are used for measuring the skin thickness?
    A. Calipers   B. Thermometer
    C. Inch tape   D. Biometer

259. What is the basic principle for treatment of obesity?
    A. Calorie reduction
    B. Increase exercise
    C. High fat intake
    D. A and B both

260. In fever the metabolism is effected as:
    A. Imbalanced   B. Balanced
    C. Both A and B   D. No effect

261. The calorie and calorie needs are measured by:
    A. Thermometer
    B. Calorimeter
    C. Biometer
    D. All of the above

262. Parotid gland is:
    A. Gastric gland   B. Intestinal gland
    C. Salivary gland   D. None of the above

263. Absorption is maximum in the small intestine because of:
    A. The presence of villi
    B. Its length
    C. Its thin walls
    D. All of the above

264. Mastication is:
    A. Digestion   B. Absorption
    C. Assimilation   D. Chewing

265. Appendix is a part of _____.
    A. Ileum   B. Duodenum
    C. Cecum   D. Colon

266. _____ secretes bile juice.
    A. Liver   B. Pancreas
    C. Salivary gland D. Intestine

267. Which of the following is chiefly digested in the stomach?
    A. Carbohydrates
    B. Proteins
    C. Fats
    D. Lipids

268. Large intestine in man mainly carries out _____.
    A. Digestion of fats B. Absorption
    C. Assimilation
    D. Digestion of carbohydrate

269. Which of the following nutrients contains the element nitrogen?
    A. Protein   B. Water
    C. Fat   D. Carbohydrates

270. Which of the following nutrients is the primary source of fuel for the body, especially the brain?
    A. Protein   B. Vitamins
    C. Carbohydrates   D. Lipids

271. _____ is the body's primary source of energy.
    A. Fructose   B. Sucrose
    C. Glycogen   D. Glucose

272. Dietary fiber is an indigestible _____ that serves separately as a body regulatory agent.
    A. Fat   B. Protein
    C. Carbohydrate   D. Amino acid

273. Overweight and obesity are major risk factors for diseases such as:
    A. Colon cancer   B. Diabetes
    C. Lung disease   D. Skin disease

274. Botulism is mainly caused due to:
    A. Mycotoxin   B. Viral toxin
    C. Bacterial toxin D. Chemical toxin

275. A whole grain is a food that has major parts:
    A. Bran, ectosperm, germ
    B. All bran, ectosperm, germ
    C. Bran, endosperm, germ
    D. Bran, endosperm, virus

276. Breaking down of larger substances into smaller units is called:
    A. Catabolism   B. Metabolism
    C. Anabolism   D. Botulism

277. The sum of body processes that change our food energy from the three energy nutrients:
   A. Anabolism   B. Catabolism
   C. Metabolism   D. Alcoholism

278. Most is reabsorbed and recycled while the rest can be trapped by fibers in the large intestine and carried out of the body with feces:
   A. Carbohydrates   B. Cholesterol
   C. Bile   D. Protein

279. In the _____, glycogen reserves protect cells from depressed metabolic function.
   A. Bile   B. Liver
   C. Small intestine D. Large intestine

280. Reserve fuel supply and basic fuel supply are the function of:
   A. Carbohydrates   B. Proteins
   C. Fats   D. Minerals

281. Functions of fat in the body:
   A. Provides a backup energy supply for the body that can be used when carbs are low
   B. Supplies essential nutrients in the form of fatty acids to the body, which are necessary for proper functioning
   C. Increases one's feeling of fullness after eating
   D. All of the above

282. _____ is essential for all metabolic processes.
   A. Vitamins   B. Water
   C. Carbohydrates   D. Proteins

283. Body protein has a source of energy of:
   A. 9 kcal/g   B. 6 kcal/g
   C. 3 kcal/g   D. 4 kcal/g

284. Digestion in the mouth and esophagus has a mechanical digestion when this breaks down food:
   A. Constipation   B. Mastication
   C. Lubrication   D. Both A and B

285. Protein is a source of:
   A. 9 kcal/g   B. 4 kcal/g
   C. 5 kcal/g   D. 6 kcal/g

286. What is another name of maize?
   A. Rice   B. Corn
   C. Wheat   D. All of the above

287. Having variety in diet means:
   A. Controlling portion size
   B. Making sure that you choose foods from each food groups
   C. Choosing foods rich in phytochemicals
   D. Choosing different types of foods within each food group.

288. Health promotion and disease prevention can be achieved by:
   A. Proper diet and exercise
   B. Observing no smoking effect
   C. Limiting alcohal intake and learning how to deal with stress
   D. All of the above

289. The RDAs (recommended dietary allowances) recommend nutrient amounts for essential nutrients:
   A. For practically all healthy people
   B. Will decrease risk of certain chronic diseases
   C. Are specified by gender and age
   D. All of the above

290. Fruits, vegetables and cereals are potent sources of:
   A. Antioxidants   B. Saturated fat
   C. Unsaturated fat D. Free radicals

291. One of the fat soluble vitamin helps in coagulation of blood:
   A. Vitamin A   B. Vitamin D
   C. Vitamin E   D. Vitamin K

292. A deficiency of thiamine (vitamin B_1) in the diet causes:
   A. Osteopenia   B. Beriberi
   C. Malnutrition   D. Scurvy

293. Iron supplements are frequently recommended for all of the following *except*:
    A. Women who are pregnant
    B. Infants and toddlers
    C. Teenage girls
    D. Post-menopausal women

294. Products that contain live microorganisms in sufficient numbers to alter intestinal microflora and promote intestinal microbial balance are known as:
    A. Antibodies   B. Porbiotics
    C. Enzymes   D. Vegetables

295. A substance needed by the body for growth, energy, repair and maintenance is:
    A. Nutrient   B. Carbohydrate
    C. Calorie   D. Fatty acid

296. All of the following are nutrients found in food *except* _____.
    A. Plasma   B. Proteins
    C. Carbohydrates   D. Vitamins

297. Diet high in saturated fats can be linked to which of the following?
    A. Kidney failure
    B. Bulimia
    C. Anorexia
    D. Cardiovascular disease

298. Amylases in saliva begin the breakdown of carbohydrates into:
    A. Fatty acids
    B. Polypeptides
    C. Amino acids
    D. Simple sugars

299. Your body needs vitamins and minerals because:
    A. They give energy
    B. They help in carrying metabolic activities
    C. They insulate body organs
    D. They withdraw heat from body

300. Food passes through the stomach directly by:
    A. The large intestine
    B. The small intestine
    C. The heart
    D. The pancreas

301. A(n) _____ is a unit of energy that indicates the amount of energy contained in food.
    A. Label
    B. Food guide pyramid
    C. Calorie
    D. Basket

302. For the first time, bacteria were observed by:
    A. WH Stanley   B. Louis Pasteur
    C. Robert Koch   D. AV Leewenhoek

303. Which of the following is a reducing sugar?
    A. Starch   B. Lactose
    C. Fructose   D. Sucrose

304. Calcium is used in human body for:
    A. Formation of bones
    B. Recovery of bicarbonate
    C. Utilization of sulfate
    D. Synthesis of amino acids

305. Most spoilage causing bacteria grow at:
    A. Acidic pH   B. Neutral pH
    C. Alkaline pH   D. At any pH

306. What are the extrinsic factors for microorganisms?
    A. pH
    B. Moisture
    C. Oxidation-reduction
    D. All of the above

307. Table sugar is:
    A. Sucrose   B. Fructose
    C. Galactose   D. Glucose

308. Coffee and tea contains stimulants:
   A. Caffeine
   B. Citric acid
   C. Theophylline
   D. All of the above

309. Sodium bicarbonate in cooking is usually used as:
   A. Alum   B. Baking powder
   C. Baking soda   D. Cream of tartar

310. The red color of tomato is due to presence of:
   A. Beta carotene B. Fructose
   C. Lycopene   D. Limonene

311. Leafy vegetables get most of their green color from:
   A. Carotene   B. Chlorophyll
   C. Mitochondria   D. Xanthophyll

312. Peppers contain:
   A. Acetic acid   B. Lycopene
   C. Capsaicin   D. Sulphuric acid

313. Table salt is:
   A. Iodine
   B. Potassium chloride
   C. Sodium chloride
   D. Sulfur

314. When onions are chopped the tears come out from eyes. This is due to presence of:
   A. Nitric acid
   B. Sulfuric acid
   C. Tartaric acid
   D. Citric acid

315. The major goal of the Green Revolution has been to:
   A. Decrease the use of modern farm machinery
   B. Decrease population growth
   C. Increase agricultural output
   D. Increase the number of traditional farms

316. The term Green Revolution is used to describe the:
   A. Tensions between developing and developed nations
   B. Heavy reliance on manual labor in agriculture
   C. Protests against environmental destruction caused by industry
   D. Development of new types of grains and new methods of growing them

317. Pasteurization involves the:
   A. Exposure of food to high temperatures for short periods to destroy harmful microorganisms.
   B. Exposure of food to heat to inactivate enzymes that cause undersirable effects in foods during storage.
   C. Fortification of foods with vitamins A and D
   D. Use of irradiation to destroy certain pathogens in foods

318. Those at greatest risk for food-borne illness include:
   A. Pregnant woman
   B. Infants and children
   C. Immunosuppressed individuals
   D. All of the above

319. Ancient methods of food preservation include:
   A. Pasteurizing and sterilizing
   B. Canning, blanching and irradiating
   C. Freezing and boiling
   D. Drying, smoking and fermenting

320. A biological method of food preservation is:
   A. Freezing   B. Drying
   C. Fermentation   D. Adding salt

321. The organisms used in the process of fermentation:
   A. Metabolize all the oxygen in food.
   B. Produce water in the food

C. Utilize all the nutrients in a food.

D. Produce products, such as acids, that inhibit the growth of other organism

322. Food can be kept for long periods of time by adding salt or sugar because these substances:

A. Make the food too acidic for spoilage to occur.

B. Bind to water, thereby making it unavailable to the microorganisms.

C. Effectively kills microorganisms

D. Dissolve the cell walls in plant foods.

323. Bacteria that can grow in the absence of oxygen are called:

A. Anerobes   B. Molds

C. Aerobes   D. Yeasts

324. _____ creates free radicals in food, which can destroy cell membranes and attack DNA and proteins, thus preventing microorganism growth.

A. Pasteurization

B. Irradiation

C. Reduction

D. All of the above

325. Salmonella bacteria usually spread via:

A. Raw meats, poultry and eggs

B. Pickled vegetables

C. Home canned vegetables

D. Raw vegetables

326. The food-borne illness organism often associated with small cuts and boils is:

A. Listeria

B. Staphylococcus

C. C. botulinum

D. Salmonella

327. Aflatoxins:

A. Are linked to cancer in animals

B. Are intentional food additives

C. Occur only in corn and peanut products

D. All of the above

328. Regulation of most food additives is the responsibility of the:

A. Centers for disease control and prevention

B. United States Department of Agricluture

C. Food and Drug Administration

D. Environmental Protection Agency

329. Vitamin C and vitamin E, BHA and BHT, and sulfites are all:

A. Antioxidants

B. Flavor enhancers

C. Antimicrobial agents

D. Incidental food additives

330. Nitrite prevents the growth of:

A. C. botulinum   B. C. perfringes

C. S. aureus   D. Yeasts

331. Substances used to preserve foods by lowering the pH are:

A. Vinegar and citric acid

B. Smoke and irradiation

C. Baking powder and soda

D. Salt and sugar

332. Solanine is:

A. Not known to be harmful to humans.

B. A naturally occurring toxin found in green potatoes

C. A naturally occurring toxin found in shellfish

D. A toxin that grows on corn and peanut products

333. The factor that is least important to control in order to limit food-illness is:

A. Presence of pesticides

B. Presence of microbes

C. Temperature of food

D. Time of incubation

334. Vitamin A is known as:

A. Retinol   B. Thiamine

C. Riboflavin   D. Ascorbic acid

335. Which refrigerant is commonly used is used in cold storage in our country?
    A. Ethylene   B. Carbide
    C. Ammonia   D. Sodium benzoate

336. Chillies are rich source of:
    A. Vitamin A
    B. Vittamin C
    C. Vitamins A and C
    D. Vitamin E

337. Yellow colored vegetables are rich source of:
    A. Vitamin A   B. Vitamin B
    C. Vitamin C   D. Vitamin D

338. Which of the following plant hormones is considered as ripen?
    A. Cytokinin   B. Retinol
    C. Ethylene   D. Iodine

339. In onion pink color is due to:
    A. Anthocyanin
    B. Carotene
    C. Xanthophyll
    D. Quercitin

340. Vitamin D is chemically known as:
    A. Retinol   B. Cobalamine
    C. Calciferol   D. Tocopherol

341. The non-nutritive substances added intentionally to food, generally in small quantities to improve its flavor, appearance, texture or storage properties:
    A. Food additive
    B. Food preservative
    C. Food solvent
    D. Photochemical

342. _____ include compounds that protect biological system against the potentially harmful effects of processes that can cause excessive oxidation.
    A. Vegetables   B. Antioxidants
    C. Carbohydrates   D. Fruits

343. _____ helps in preventing degenerative diseases
    A. Toxins and sulphates
    B. Additives and preservatives
    C. Phytochemicals and antioxidants
    D. Aldehydes and aflatoxins

344. The term _____ refers to covering a food with a layer of crumbs flour or other fine substances before cooking it.
    A. Coating   B. Roasting
    C. Blanching   D. Marinating

345. Passing a food through a fine dry or powdery substance in order to coat it:
    A. Battering   B. Breading
    C. Dredging   D. None of the above

346. Plunging food into boiling liquid and immersing in cold water:
    A. Marinating
    B. Fermentation
    C. Grinding
    D. Blanching

347. _____ is a process of breaking down of complex matter into simpler ones with aid of enzyme and bacteria.
    A. Fermentation   B. Grinding
    C. Roasting   D. Drying

348. _____ is cooling foods by just immersing them in water at 100 °C.
    A. Boiling   B. Poaching
    C. Simmering   D. Stewing

349. This involves cooking in the minimum amount of liquid at a temperature of 80–85 °C.
    A. Simmering   B. Poaching
    C. Stewing   D. Boiling

350. This method requires the food to be cooked in steam:
    A. Boiling   B. Steaming
    C. Poaching   D. Stewing

351. _____ consists of placing the food below or above or in between a red hot surface.

A. Grilling or boiling

B. Baking

C. Pan broiling or roasting

D. Sauteing

352. Compared to water food is cooked _____ is fat.

A. Slowing   B. Quicker

C. Same time   D. None of the above

353. _____ is a combined method of roasting and stewing in a pan with a tight fitting lid.

A. Stewing   B. Braising

C. Broiling   D. Sauteing

354. _____ from a power source magnetron are absorbed by the food and food becomes hot at once.

A. Broiling

B. Microwave cooking

C. Braising

D. Solar cooking

355. The outer layer, epidermis of the cereal consists of thin walled long rectangular cells:

A. Bran

B. Endosperm

C. Aleurone cell layer

D. Embryo

356. Botanically wheat is called:

A. *Oryzus sativus*

B. *Magnifera indica*

C. *Triticum aestivum*

D. *Brassica sarson*

357. Soaking paddy in water for a short time followed by heating once or twice in steam and drying before milling:

A. Parboiling   B. Fermentation

C. Milling   D. Germination

358. The yolk of the egg is enclosed in a sac called the:

A. Vitelline membrane

B. Plasma

C. Cuticle

D. Lipovitellinin

359. Dry heat also brings changes to starch granules through a process known as:

A. Fermentation

B. Syneresis

C. Retrogradation

D. Dextrinization

360. Aflatoxins are produced by:

A. Salmonella

B. Staphylococcus

C. C. Botulinum

D. *Aspergillus falvus*

361. _____ enzyme is secreted by the young calves brings about coagulation of milk.

A. Xanthine oxidase B. Lysine

C. Rennin   D. Carboxy amylase

362. Tea comes from which plant:

A. *Coffee thea*

B. *Ibex paraquasensis*

C. *Camelia sinesis*

D. *Camelis japonica*

363. Fenugreek is an essential spice in:

A. Curry   B. Pasta

C. Spice   D. Noodles

364. The biological value of foods is based on which main nutrient:

A. Carbohydrates   B. Fats

C. Proteins   D. Fiber

365. Carotenoids are popular food colors. In which natural product(s) do they mainly occur?

A. Grapes   B. Meat

C. Oranges   D. Beetroot

366. **What is the name for health-improving bacteria added to our food (like in dairy products)?**

    A. Probiotics   B. Prebiotics
    C. Synbiotics   D. Symbiotics

367. **The fuzzy or cottony appearance growth on food indicates that:**

    A. Yeasts   B. Molds
    C. Bacteria   D. None of the above

368. **_____ is primarily present in the intracellular fluid (about 12.6 g/kg) in the body.**

    A. Sodium   B. Potassium
    C. Magnesium   D. Chlorine

369. **Abnormal dryness on skin and eye is called:**

    A. Blindness   B. Xerosis
    C. Cheilosis   D. Anemia

370. **_____ is also known as erythrocytes.**

    A. Red blood cells   B. White blood cells
    C. Platelets   D. Plasma

371. **The fluid portion of blood in which formed cells (white blood cells, red blood cells, platelets) are suspended:**

    A. Serum   B. Platelets
    C. Plasma   D. Hemoglobin

372. **Bleeding and swollen gums are the signs of:**

    A. Pellagra   B. Anemia
    C. Rickets   D. Scurvy

373. **The undesirable change in a food that makes it unsafe for human consumption is referred to as:**

    A. Food decay   B. Food loss
    C. Food spoilage   D. All of the above

374. **Food preservation involves:**

    A. Increasing shelf life
    B. Ensuring safety for human consumption

    C. Both A and B
    D. All of the above

375. **Pasteurization is:**

    A. Low temperature treatment
    B. Steaming treatment
    C. High temperature treatment
    D. Low and high temperature treatment

376. **Which of the following statement is true about chemical preservative?**

    A. Microbial or microstatic agents
    B. Chemical preservatives often hazardous to humans
    C. Sodium benzoate is widely used preservative
    D. All of the above

377. **Botulinum is caused by:**

    A. *Clostridium botulinum*
    B. All *Clostridium* species
    C. *Clostridium tetani*
    D. *Clostridium subtilis*

378. **Which of the following is true about botulinal poisoning?**

    A. Is a neurotoxin
    B. Water soluble exotoxin
    C. Is produced by *Clostridium botulinum*
    D. All of the above

379. **Starches are major components of:**

    A. Vegetables   B. Fruits
    C. Cereals   D. All of the above

380. **Sugar, starch, pectins and gums are the major _____ found in foods.**

    A. Proteins   B. Fats
    C. Minerals   D. Carbohydrates

381. **The primary protein in milk is:**

    A. Casein   B. Tryptophan
    C. Lysine   D. Arginine

382. **The primary milk carbohydrate is:**

    A. Leucine   B. Sucrose
    C. Arginine   D. Lactose

383. Which of the following is an example of physical digestion?

A. The chewing of food into smaller pieces in the mouth

B. The killing of bacteria in food in the stomach

C. The digestion of food by enzymes in the stomach

D. The changing of starch into maltose in the mouth

384. Which one of the following is not a function of water in the human body?

A. Helps eliminate wastes

B. It regulates body temperature

C. Helps in the formation of bones

D. It transports nutrients around the body

385. Which of the following food types passes through the digestive system without being used up?

A. Vitamins B. Minerals

C. Fiber D. Starch

386. Where in the body is bile produced?

A. The small intestine

B. The pancreas

C. The liver

D. The kidneys

387. This type of nutrient acts as an energy store and also acts as an insulator:

A. Minerals B. Water

C. Fat D. Fiber

388. _____ is the basic nutrient needed for growth, maintenance and replacement of body cells and forms hormones and enzymes which regulate body processes.

A. Proteins B. Carbohydrates

C. Fats D. Vitamins

389. The basic nutrient supplies energy and fiber:

A. Protein B. Carbohydrates

C. Fats D. Minerals

390. Which of the following seems to be the causal agent of peptic ulcers?

A. *Helicobacter pylori*

B. *Salmonella typhi*

C. Hepatitis A virus

D. *Campylobacter jejuni*

391. The process of digestion of food in humans begins in:

A. Stomach B. Food pipe

C. Mouth D. Small intestine

392. The process of digestion in humans is completed in:

A. Esophagus B. Small intestine

C. Stomach D. Large intestine

393. In human digestive system, bile is secreted by:

A. Pancreas B. Liver

C. Kidneys D. Stomach

394. The correct order of steps occurring in nutrition in animals is:

A. Ingestion → Absorption → Digestion → Assimilation

B. Ingestion → Digestion → Assimilation → Absorption

C. Ingestion → Digestion → Absorption → Assimilation

D. Ingestion → Assimilation → Digestion → Absorption

395. In human digestive system, the enzymes pepsin and trypsin are secreted respectively by:

A. Pancreas and liver

B. Stomach and salivary glands

C. Pancreas and gallbladder

D. Stomach and pancreas

396. Which of the following is the correct statement regarding bile?

A. Secreted by bile duct and stored in liver

B. Secreted by gallbladder and stored in liver

C. Secreted by liver and stored in bile duct

D. Secreted by liver and stored in gall-bladder

397. Where are proteins first digested in the alimentary canal?

A. Small intestine B. Esophagus

C. Mouth D. Stomach

398. The inner lining of stomach is protected by one of the following from the harmful effect of hydrochloric acid. This is:

A. Pepsin B. Mucus

C. Saliva D. Bile

399. Which part of alimentary canal receives bile from the liver?

A. Small intestine

B. Oesophagus

C. Stomach

D. Large intestine

400. Which of the following component of our food is digested by an enzyme, which is present in saliva as well as in pancreatic juice?

A. Proteins B. Fat

C. Minerals D. Carbohydrate

401. If the saliva is lacking in salivary amylase, then which of the following processes taking place in the buccal cavity will be affected?

A. Proteins breaking down into amino acids

B. Starch breaking down into sugars

C. Fats breaking down into fatty acids and glycerol

D. Intestinal layer breaking down leading to ulcers

402. Which of the following is the correct functions of two components of pancreatic juice trypsin and lipase?

A. Trypsin digests proteins and lipase carbohydrates

B. Trypsin digests emulsified fats and lipase proteins

C. Trypsin digests starch and lipase fats

D. Trypsin digests proteins and lipase emulsified fats

403. Which of the following is the correct sequence of parts as they occur in the human alimentary canal?

A. Mouth → Stomach → Small intestine → Esophagus → Large intestine

B. Mouth → Esophagus → Stomach → Large intestine → Small intestine

C. Mouth → Stomach → Esophagus → Small intestine → Large intestine

D. Mouth → Esophagus → Stomach → Small intestine → Large intestine

404. Which of the following best describes food preservation?

A. The storage of food for future use

B. The addition of chemical preservatives to prevent spoilage by microorganisms

C. The making of jams and jellies

D. The packaging of food in air tight containers

405. What is the reason for dehydrating food?

A. To make the food crispy

B. To make the food light

C. To make the food brown in color

D. To remove moisture from the food

406. At 9 calories per gram, which is the most concentrated source of energy?

A. Proteins B. Carbohydrates

C. Vitamins D. Fats

407. Which of the following is not a function of fiber?

A. It supplies the body with energy

B. It regulates bowel functions

C. It reduces the risk of intestinal problems

D. It promotes the feeling of fullness

408. Which vitamin is known to help construct DNA as well as prevent birth defects?

A. Magnesium B. Folic acid

C. Potassium D. Copper

409. Which of the following is not a function of water?
    A. It transports nutrients
    B. It cushions organs
    C. It maintains body temperature
    D. It fuels the body

410. The nutritive value of cereals is effected by:
    A. Processing   B. Milling
    C. Cooking   D. All of the above

411. Which of the following is small molecules directly absorbed by the small intestine without digestion?
    A. Fiber   B. Starch
    C. Sugar   D. Fat

412. Small amounts of minerals and vitamins are needed for good health and vitality. Which of the following part of our diet is needed for nerve function?
    A. Fluorine   B. Vitamin C
    C. Sodium   D. Calcium

413. Which is not a symptom of diabetes mellitus?
    A. Polycythemia   B. Polyphagia
    C. Polydypsia   D. Polyuria

414. What is the name of the hormone which decreases blood glucose?
    A. Glucagon   B. Insulin
    C. Melatonin   D. Seratonin

415. Which is not a symptom of diabetes mellitus?
    A. Polyuria   B. Polycythemia
    C. Polyphagia   D. Polydypsia

416. Medical term for high blood pressure is:
    A. Hyperglycemia   B. Hyperuricemia
    C. Hypertension   D. Hyperthyroidism

417. What unit is used to measure the blood pressure in clinical practice?
    A. mg/dl   B. mbar
    C. mmHg   D. Calorie

418. What unit is used to measure blood sugar?
    A. mg/dl   B. mbar
    C. mmHg   D. Calorie

419. Casein is classified as phosphoprotein because of presence of:
    A. Lactose   B. Albumin
    C. Phosphoric acid   D. Maltose

420. White color of milk is due to presence of:
    A. Casein   B. Calcium
    C. Phosphorus   D. All of the above

421. Milk is slightly sweet because of presence of:
    A. Casein   B. Vitamin C
    C. Carotene   D. Lactose

422. Milk is poor source of:
    A. Vitamin C   B. Iron
    C. Both A and B   D. None of the above

423. The rapid darkening of the cut surface of apple, brinjal, potato, and banana are examples of:
    A. Maillard reaction
    B. Enzymatic browning reaction
    C. Dextrinization
    D. None of the above

424. Spoilage of fats is called:
    A. Viscosity   B. Rancidity
    C. Acidity   D. All of the above

425. Functions of spices in food are:
    A. Adds flavor and color
    B. Stimulates salivation
    C. Antibacterial and antifungal
    D. All of the above

426. What did Louis Pasteur invent in the 1860s?
    A. Skimming treatment
    B. Heat treatment
    C. Whipping treatment
    D. Pasteurized treatment

427. **What dairy product contains several nutrients?**
    A. Milk   B. Ice cream
    C. Cream   D. Cheese

428. **What two vitamins does milk contain?**
    A. A and C
    B. A and D
    C. E and C
    D. C and D

429. **What creates buttermilk?**
    A. Whipped cream mixed with milk
    B. Slightly sweetened melted butter
    C. Butter mixed in with milk
    D. The watery portion of cream

430. **Almonds are found to have beneficial effect on:**
    A. Anemia
    B. Cardiovascular diseases
    C. Skeletal problems
    D. All of the above

431. **During emulsification, bile salts break down _____ globules into smaller fat droplets.**
    A. Fat   B. Liquid
    C. Proteins   D. Vitamins

432. **_____ is a chemical secreted by the small intestine.**
    A. Enzymes   B. Bile
    C. Fats   D. Proteins

433. **The liver stores fat-soluble nutrients and regulates the level of _____ molecules in the blood.**
    A. Vitamins
    B. Proteins
    C. Food
    D. Chemicals

434. **The skin can be considered an _____ organ.**
    A. Lipid   B. Endocrine
    C. Respiratory   D. Excretory

435. **The blood-cleaning units of the kidneys are called _____.**
    A. Nephrons   B. Dialysis
    C. Salts   D. Liver

436. **Dialysis is a _____ solution to kidney failure.**
    A. Temporarily   B. Permanent
    C. Unpleasant   D. None of the above

437. **Which of the following is considered nutrients?**
    A. Lipids   B. Proteins
    C. Both A and B   D. None of the above

438. **Nutrients provide the body with the energy and materials, it needs for _____.**
    A. Growth   B. Maintenance
    C. Repair   D. All of the above

439. **Most of the body's energy needs should be supplied by dietary_____.**
    A. Carbohydrates   B. Fats
    C. Vitamins   D. Proteins

440. **A _____ is a substance needed by the body for growth, energy, repair, and maintenance.**
    A. Carbohydrates
    B. Lipids
    C. Calorie
    D. Nutrient

441. **Consumption of khesari dal leads to:**
    A. Lathyrism   B. Anemia
    C. Dropsy   D. Kala-azar

442. **Entropy means:**
    A. Conservation   B. Creation
    C. Growth   D. Disorder

443. **ORS stands for:**
    A. Oral recharging solution
    B. Oral reducing solution
    C. Oral rehydration solution
    D. Oral replenishing solution

444. Ragi is a richest source of:
- A. Iron
- B. Calcium
- C. Vitamin C
- D. Iodine

445. The lifespan of a human RBC is:
- A. One day
- B. One week
- C. One month
- D. Four months

446. Nitrogen is secreted by humans in form of:
- A. Ammonia
- B. Urea
- C. Uric acid
- D. Amino acid

447. Cereals are mainly rich in:
- A. Starch
- B. Proteins
- C. Vitamin C
- D. Minerals

448. Which of the following is a vitamin?
- A. Insulin
- B. Calcium
- C. Retinol
- D. Lipase

449. _____ test is used for detection of typhoid.
- A. Liver function test
- B. Hemoglobin test
- C. Widal test
- D. All of the above

450. Amnesia is related to loss:
- A. Memory
- B. Blood
- C. Oxygen
- D. Energy

451. Roughage, a necessary constituent of diet, consists largely of indigestible:
- A. Carbohydrates such as cellulose and lignin
- B. Carbohydrates (cellulose and lignin) and unsaturated fatty acids
- C. Carbohydrates (cellulose and lignin) and semi-cooked meat
- D. All of the above

452. In human beings fats are stored in:
- A. Epithelial tissues
- B. Red blood cells
- C. Adipose tissue
- D. Gallbladder

453. Which of the following seeds are found to be beneficial for diabetic patient?
- A. Cumin seeds
- B. Fenugreek seeds
- C. Mustard seeds
- D. Aniseed

454. Botulism caused by *Clostridium botulinum* affects the:
- A. Heart
- B. Liver
- C. Neuromuscular junction
- D. Spleen

455. High level of iron in body leads to:
- A. Anemia
- B. Hemochromatosis
- C. Diabetes mellitus
- D. Salmonella

456. A function of carbohydrates in the diet is to:
- A. Provide energy
- B. Maintain fluid balance
- C. Promote growth, maintenance and repair
- D. Stimulate chemical reactions in body

457. An individual who has met specified educational and experience criteria by the state licensing board to be considered a nutrition expert:
- A. Nutritionist
- B. Registered dietitian
- C. Licensed dietitian
- D. Nutrition educator

458. The energy-yielding nutrient with the highest caloric content is:
- A. Fat
- B. Protein
- C. Carbohydrate
- D. Mineral

459. Nutritional genomic is concerned with:
- A. Family health histories
- B. Relationship of nutrition and gene expression

C. Promoting access to healthful foods

D. Eliminating chronic diseases

460. **The nutrient that helps to maintain hydration and body temperature is:**

A. Protein

B. Water

C. Carbohydrates

D. Vitamin

461. **The nutrient that acts as a lubricant and protective cushion is:**

A. Protein   B. Mineral

C. Carbohydrate   D. Water

462. **The nutrient that acts as insulation under the skin to help maintain body temperature is:**

A. Fat   B. Protein

C. Carbohydrate   D. Water

463. **A high fiber food includes:**

A. Fruit juice

B. Ice cream

C. Carbonated beverage

D. Whole grains

464. **Which part is the protective coating that surrounds the grain?**

A. Hull   B. Bran

C. Germ   D. Endosperm

465. **Which of these statements about bacteria is true?**

A. All types of bacteria give food poisoning

B. Freezing makes food last longer by killing bacteria

C. Bacteria grow fastest when they are warm

D. All bacteria need air to survive

466. **Which one of the food is liked to contain most bacteria?**

A. Cooked chicken

B. Tinned cream

C. Frozen raw chicken

D. Bottled mayonnaise

467. **At work place the best way to dry your hands is:**

A. Using a warm air dryer

B. Give them a shake

C. Using a cotton towel

D. Using a paper towel

468. **Food contaminated with food poisoning bacteria would:**

A. Smell

B. Change color

C. Look and taste normal

D. Be slimy and bitter

469. **Food poisoning only occurs because of bad practice in:**

A. Restaurants

B. Retail shops

C. Home and domestic kitchens

D. All of the above

470. **What does vitamin K deficiency lead to?**

A. Problem in digestion

B. Problem in blood coagulation

C. Problem in calcium metabolism

D. All the the above

471. **What is the condition known as, in which the body does not get its fair share of nutrients, either from starvation, or as a result of poor absorption?**

A. Marasmus

B. Malnutrition

C. Kwashiorkor

D. Malnutrition and marasmus

472. **Kwashiorkor disease is caused due to the deficiency of:**

A. Lysine

B. Unsaturated fatty acids

C. Vitamin K

D. Protein

473. The weight gain (in gram) per gram protein consumed is called:

A. Net protein ratio (NPR)

B. Biological value

C. Protein efficiency ratio

D. Chemical scores

474. Which of the following statements is not correct in relation to muscle proteins?

A. Actin and myosin interact to form actomyosin which is responsible for muscle contraction

B. Collagen contributes to the toughness of muscles due to its abundant presence

C. Elastin, a constituent of ligaments, is tougher than collagen

D. Actomyosin is not the main state of actin and myosin in postmortem muscles

475. Diabetes is a:

A. Metabolic disorder

B. Digestive disorder

C. Mental disorder

D. All of the above

476. Anorexia nervosa is:

A. Psychological disorder

B. Eating disorder

C. Both A and B

D. None of the above

477. The percentage of protein in milk is:

A. 1–2%   B. 3–4%

C. 5–6%   D. 7–8%

478. The main component of protein is:

A. Hydrogen

B. Nitrogen

C. Oxygen

D. Carbon

479. Our food is divided into how many groups?

A. Three   B. Two

C. One   D. None of the above

480. The working capacity during illness:

A. Increases

B. Decreases

C. Not affected

D. None of the above

481. The protein requirement of infant in comparison to adult is:

A. More   B. Very less

C. Less   D. Not required

482. When the calorie requirement of infant are not fullfilled, the weight:

A. Increases

B. Increases slowly

C. Remains same

D. Increases rapidly

483. Natural source of getting vitamin D is:

A. Sunrays   B. Fire

C. Water   D. Air

484. The vitamin which is required for development of bones for infant is:

A. Vitamin A   B. Vitamin B

C. Vitamin C   D. Vitamin D

485. _____ is important for the formation of bones and teeth.

A. Calcium   B. Iron

C. Vitamin A   D. Vitamin C

486. Difference in growth and development is observed during _____ age.

A. During 5 years

B. During 10 years

C. During 8 years

D. During 6 years

487. Malabsorption types are:

A. 4   B. 3

C. 1   D. 5

488. Poached egg are prepared in:

A. In oil

B. In ghee and water

C. In butter

D. All of the above

489. In body the % of water remains in liquid form in cells is:

  A. 50%   B. 25%

  C. 70%   D. 20%

490. Death occurs when the % of water decreases up to:

  A. 50%   B. 20%

  C. 10%   D. 40%

491. Vitamin was invented by:

  A. Funk   B. Leunin

  C. Thomas   D. Mendel

492. Vitamin B$_1$ is taken during:

  A. Daytime   B. Night

  C. Afternoon   D. Evening

493. During pregnancy the deficiency of calcium in fetus leads to:

  A. Osteomalacia

  B. Malnutrition

  C. Anemia

  D. None of the above

494. Vitamin D is necessary for absorption of

  A. Fluorine   B. Calcium

  C. Sodium   D. Potassium

495. Heme iron is found in:

  A. Hemoglobin   B. Myoglobin

  C. Both A and B   D. None of the above

496. Who said healthy mind lies in healthy body:

  A. Aristotle

  B. Eudkin

  C. Tewer

  D. Herbart and Spencer

497. From birth till death complete food, is:

  A. Food grains   B. Vegetables

  C. Milk   D. Fruits

498. Animal foods are:

  A. Egg, bread, biscuit

  B. Meat, fish and egg

  C. Pulses, fruits and vegetables

  D. None of the above

499. Iron absorption is enhanced in body by intake of _____ vitamin.

  A. Vitamin A   B. Vitamin B

  C. Vitamin C   D. Vitamin D

500. In lactating mother about _____ liters of milk is produced.

  A. 1/2 liter   B. 1 liter

  C. 1.5 liter   D. 2 liter

501. Which of these methods of cooking with fat uses the least amount of fat?

  A. Stir-frying

  B. Deep frying

  C. Sauteing

  D. Boiling

502. Convenience foods:

  A. Usually cost less than the same foods made from scratch

  B. require a long time for preparation

  C. Tend to contain more fat, sugar and salt than foods made from scratch

  D. They are poisonous

503. An agency of India engaged in periodic diet and nutrition surveys is:

  A. ICAR (Indian Council of Agricultural Research)

  B. NNMB (National Nutrition Monitoring Bureau)

  C. WHO (World Health Organization)

  D. FAO (Food and Agricultural Organization)

504. _____ is the residue that remains after sucrose crystals have been removed from the concentrated juices of sugar.

  A. Ash   B. Moisture

  C. Molasses   D. Water

505. Jaggery is mainly obtained from:
   A. Beet root   B. Sweet potato
   C. Tomato   D. Sugarcane

506. Preservation of Food Adulteration Act (PFA) classifies preservatives as:
   A. Class I preservatives
   B. Class II preservatives
   C. Both a and b
   D. None of the above

507. Class I preservatives are:
   A. Salt and sugar
   B. Spices and vinegar
   C. Honey and vegetable oils
   D. All of the above

508. Class II preservatives are:
   A. Benzoic acid
   B. Sodium and potassium salts
   C. Both a and b
   D. None of the above

509. Removal of water from a product while it is frozen by sublimation is called:
   A. Sun drying   B. Freeze drying
   C. Spray drying   D. Smoking

510. The word combining nutrition and pharmaceuticals refers to:
   A. Nutraceuticals
   B. Nutriceuticals
   C. Nutritionceuticals
   D. New pharmaceuticals

511. Food contamination can occur during:
   A. Food preparation
   B. Serving
   C. Cooking
   D. All of the above

512. Most food-borne illnesses go undiagnosed because:
   A. Most victims die before treatment
   B. The symptoms are not serious enough to warrant a hospital visit
   C. Symptoms usually appear during flu season
   D. Symptoms may not appear for a week or more

513. In order to survive and multiply, all bacteria require:
   A. Food, moisture, proper pH, and proper temperature
   B. Food, proper temperature and time
   C. Food, moisture, proper pH, proper temperature and time
   D. Food, moisture, and proper pH

514. The hepatitis A virus is:
   A. Transmitted by poor personal hygiene
   B. Often caused by contaminated shellfish
   C. Carried by humans
   D. All of the above

515. Toxic metal contamination can occur through:
   A. Shellfish harvested from waters with high levels of mercury or lead
   B. Cooking acidic foods, such as tomatoes, in an unlined copper pan
   C. Serving foods in lead glazed ceramics
   D. All of the above

516. HACCP is a system for:
   A. Maintaining food safety
   B. Controlling cooking quality
   C. Standardizing recipes
   D. Controlling the food costs

517. Cross-contamination can be reduced by:
   A. Personal cleanliness and hygiene
   B. Labeling all food items
   C. Reducing the time that food is in the danger zone
   D. All of the above

518. A food-borne illness caused by _____ would be considered an infection.
   A. Mercury   B. Melamine
   C. Bacteria   D. Insecticides

519. Which of the following can be used to inhibit bacterial growth?

A. High levels of sugar

B. High levels of salt

C. Dehydration

D. All of the above

520. Which of the following is a bad food handling practice?

A. Cleaning cutting boards and knives thoroughly after using with fresh meat

B. Storing cooked and fresh meat in the same container

C. Prompt refrigeration of fresh and cooked foods in separate containers

D. Thoroughly cooking poultry before eating

521. A physician should be consulted for which of the following symptoms of diarrheal illness?

A. Temperature of 98.6 °F

B. Blood in stool

C. Upset stomach

D. Diarrhea lasting one day

522. Roots and tubers are poor source of:

A. Calcium   B. Iron

C. Protein   D. All of the above

523. The following list describes four major digestive enzymes. Which one of the following is incorrect?

A. Salivary amylase-salivary glands-mouth

B. Pepsin-gastric glands-stomach

C. Nuclease-small intestine-stomach

D. Lipase-pancreas-small intestine

524. Which of the following would be the best advice for reducing nutrition-related health risks?

A. Avoid artificial preservatives and colors

B. Eat a variety of foods

C. Eat energy dense foods

D. Choose organically grown fruits and vegetables

525. The most likely cause of food-related health risk is:

A. Food additives

B. Toxicants

C. Environmental contaminants

D. Microbial contamination

526. Which of the following is not normally considered to be a food additive?

A. Salt

B. Artificial sweeteners

C. Antioxidants

D. Artificial color

527. Organic foods are:

A. Grown without the use of synthetic chemicals such as pesticides and fertilizers

B. Free of pesticide residues and other contaminants

C. Distinct to other foods as they contain only natural ingredients

D. All of the above

528. Water activity relates to:

A. Water in food which is available to allow microorganism growth

B. The rate of osmosis into the microbial cells

C. The water bound to food particles

D. Salt concentration of food

529. The HACCP system involves:

A. Identification of processes in food production where the risk of contamination is high

B. Development and implementation of a plan to control identified risks

C. Immediately acting to correct identified hazards

D. All of the above

530. Nutritional status assessment involves consideration of which of the following data?

A. Clinical and laboratory

B. Psychosocial and demographic

C. Anthropometry and diet history

D. All of the above

531. Which nutrient is the best energy source for your body?

A. Carbohydrates

B. Proteins

C. Minerals

D. Fats

532. Which nutrient is most important for building and repairing the cells in your body?

A. Carbohydrates

B. Proteins

C. Vitamins

D. Fats

533. Which mineral is most important for keeping bones strong and healthy?

A. Zinc

B. Sodium

C. Calcium

D. Magnesium

534. Why are fats important for a healthy body?

A. Fats store vitamins A, D, and E

B. Fats are part of your brain and nerves

C. Fat helps keep you warm

D. All of the above

535. The word calorie is best related to which word?

A. Fat

B. Energy

C. Protein

D. Serving

536. What does your body do with calories you eat but do not use?

A. Gets rid of them

B. Your body always uses all the calories you eat

C. Stores unused calories as fat

D. All of the above

537. This is a basic rule of healthy eating—eat a _____ of food.

A. Lot

B. Variety

C. Pound

D. Mouthful

538. During fasting, in what sequence the following body nutrients are utilized:

A. Fats-carbohydrates-proteins

B. Carbohydrates-proteins-lipids

C. Proteins-carbohydrates-fats

D. Carbohydrates-fats-proteins

539. In protein deficiency if symptoms like thin limbs, related growth of body and brain, edema, diarrhea, etc. develop the disease are called:

A. Pellagra

B. Kwashiorkor

C. Marasmus

D. Anemia

540. Xerophthalmia in man is caused by deficiency of:

A. Vitamin K

B. Vitamin A

C. Vitamin C

D. Vitamin D

541. The science concerned with vegetable culture is called:

A. Floriculture

B. Olericulture

C. Horticulture

D. Agriculture

542. Which of the following elements is almost nonessential for plants?

A. Ca

B. Mo

C. Zn

D. Na

543. Bioherbicides have been recommended:

A. To prevent ecodegradation

B. Because of their ready availability

C. Because of their cheap rates

D. Because of their abundance

544. Honey is a:

A. Protein

B. Carbohydrate

C. Fat

D. None of the above

545. Which of the following is not one of the primary responsibilities of a director of food and beverage?

A. Training

B. Budgeting

C. Marketing

D. Exceeding guest expectations

546. If soap and running water are not available to clean your hands, which of the following is the best temporary alternative:
   A. Alcohol-based hand sanitizer
   B. A clean hand towel
   C. A basin filled with water
   D. None of the above

547. Which of the following is a food infection?
   A. Salmonellosis
   B. Botulism
   C. Staphylococcal intoxication
   D. None of the above

548. Which of the following minerals has not been yet proven to be essential to human biochemical systems?
   A. Selenium   B. Molybdenum
   C. Fluorine   D. Arsenic

549. Dairy foods are major sources of:
   A. Iron   B. Calcium
   C. Vitamin C   D. Selenium

550. The process by which the nutrients are added to foods to maintain the quality of diet of community is called:
   A. Emulsification
   B. Food selection
   C. Food fortification
   D. Extrusion

551. In _____, the shape of the red blood cells is altered to sickle shape.
   A. Sickle cell anemia
   B. Hemochromatosis
   C. Erythropoietic porphyria
   D. Hyperoxaluria

552. Partial discoloration in the skin, a condition caused when a person's melanocyte is not able to produce melanin, is:
   A. Albinism
   B. Vitiligo
   C. Incontinentia pigmenti
   D. SADAN

553. Largest endocrine gland of the body is:
   A. Liver   B. Thyroid
   C. Adrenal   D. Pituitary

554. Gland of the body having both endocrine and exocrine secretion:
   A. Testis   B. Ovary
   C. Pancreas   D. Stomach

555. Hyposecretion of ADH (antidiuretic hormone or vasopressin) is responsible for the disease:
   A. Diabetes insipidus
   B. Diabetes mellitus
   C. Acromicria
   D. Acromegaly

556. The synthesis of which hormone depends on the dietary intake of iodine by a person?
   A. Thyroxin
   B. Prolactin
   C. Follicle stimulating hormone (FSH)
   D. Leuteinizing hormone (LH)

557. Hyposecretion of growth hormone in adult causes:
   A. Acromicria   B. Acromegaly
   C. Dwarfism   D. Gigantism

558. Diabetes mellitus is disease caused by the hyposecretion of:
   A. Insulin   B. Glucagon
   C. Somatostatin   D. ADH

559. Male gonads are called:
   A. Testes   B. Blastocyst
   C. Ovaries   D. Scrotal sac

560. The fertilized egg is called:
   A. Ovum   B. Diploid cells
   C. Sperm   D. Zygote

561. Female gonads are called:
   A. Sperm   B. Ovary
   C. Diploid cells   D. None of the above

562. The attachment of embryo to the uterus is called:

A. Gestation   B. Fertilization

C. Implantation   D. Menstruation

563. The first time that the monthly bleeding occurs is called:

A. Maturity   B. Menarche

C. Menopause   D. Puberty

564. The lining or inner layer of the uterus is called the:

A. Cervix   B. Vagina

C. Myocardium   D. Endometrium

565. In humans, fertilization of an egg normally takes place when the sperm and egg unite in the:

A. Vagina   B. Uterus

C. Fallopian tube   D. Ovary

566. In the female reproductive system sperms follow the following route:

A. Vagina-cervical canal-fallopian tube-uterus

B. Vagina-cervical canal-uterus-fallopian tube

C. Vagina-fallopian tube-cervical canal-uterus

D. None of the above

567. All of the following diseases are caused by virus except:

A. Jaundice   B. Enfluenza

C. Typhoid   D. Mumps

568. Prothrombin, which is useful in the coagulation of blood is manufactured in?

A. Heart   B. Kidney

C. Liver   D. Stomach

569. Chickenpox is caused by:

A. Varicella virus

B. Adenovirus

C. Bacteriophage T2

D. SV40 virus

570. The stomach does not digest itself because:

A. The stomach wall is not composed of protein and so there is no digestive enzyme to attack it

B. The digestive enzyme in stomach are not efficient enough

C. The stomach wall is protected by copious amount of mucus

D. None of the above

571. Radish is a:

A. Bulb   B. Corn

C. Modified root   D. Tuber

572. The wheat kernel consists of the following:

A. Bran, germ, and endosperm

B. Bran, husk, and germ

C. Germ, husk, and bran

D. All of the above

573. BCG issued to prevent:

A. Hydrophobia   B. Cancer

C. Tuberculosis   D. Neuroglia

574. _____ is the hard outer covering of kernel.

A. Bran   B. Germ

C. Endosperm   D. None of the above

575. Whey proteins are made up of:

A. α-lactalbumin

B. β-lactalbumin

C. Both of these

D. None of the above

576. Fresh milk has a pH of about:

A. 6.5–6.7   B. 8.5–8.7

C. 5.5–5.6   D. 4.5–6.5

577. Probiotics are called:

A. Cancer inducing microbes

B. Safe antibiotics

C. New kind of food allergens

D. Live microbial food supplement

578. Excessive loss of water from tissues of the body:

   A. Rehydration

   B. Ascites

   C. Dehydration

   D. All of the above

579. _____ is a process by which the food is taken inside the body of an organism.

   A. Digestion   B. Excretion

   C. Ingestion   D. Assimilation

580. The process through which the undigested food is removed from the body is:

   A. Egestion   B. Ingestion

   C. Assimilation   D. Absorption

581. The absorbed simple soluble food substances are transported to the different parts of the body where they are utilized by the body for energy, growth and repair this process is called:

   A. Egestion   B. Ingestion

   C. Assimilation   D. Absorption

582. It is ensured that the flavor of the food is retained because:

   A. Stimulates digestive juices secretions

   B. Aids effective digestion

   C. Helps assimilation of foods

   D. All of the above

583. The properties of starch are:
   i. Bland in taste
   ii. Not readily soluble in water
   iii. Absorbs water when soaked in cold water
   iv. With cold water form temporary suspension

   A. i, ii, iii, iv   B. i, ii, iii

   C. i, ii   D. i, iv

584. Bottled milk exposed to strong sunlight lose _____ vitamin.

   A. Protein   B. Fat

   C. Riboflavin   D. Carbohydrate

585. The flavor of fruits are affected by:

   A. Sugar   B. Tannins

   C. Mineral salts   D. All of the above

586. Qualities of food affected by fortification:
   i. Flavor
   ii. Appearance
   iii. Cooking properties
   iv. Cost

   A. i, ii, iii, iv   B. i, ii, iii

   C. i, ii   D. i, iv

587. Bacteria vary in their requirement of:
   i. Food
   ii. Moisture
   iii. pH
   iv. Temperature and oxygen

   A. i, ii, iii, iv   B. i, ii, iii

   C. i, ii   D. i, iv

588. Lower temperature for a longer time in drying process:
   i. Better quality
   ii. Better retention of vitamin
   iii. Crisp
   iv. Brittle

   A. i, ii, iii, iv   B. i, ii, iii

   C. i, ii   D. i, iv

589. Preservation of food in sealed containers involving applications of heat:

   A. Dehydration   B. Canning

   C. Sterilization   D. Pasteurization

590. The heating process in canning brings about:
   i. Food cooking
   ii. Change in physical nature
   iii. Flavor and appearance change
   iv. Activity of enzymes

   A. i, ii, iii, iv   B. i, ii, iii

   C. i, ii   D. i, iv

591. Which of factors should be examined in canning process?
   i. Selection of food
   ii. Sterilization of can

iii. Sealing of cans

iv. Storage

  A. i, ii, iii, iv   B. i, ii, iii

  C. i, ii   D. i, iv

592. Canning method of preservation is applicable to:

  i. Fruit juices

  ii. Syrups

  iii. Sauces

  iv. Fruit products

  A. i, ii, iii, iv   B. i, ii, iii

  C. i, ii   D. i, iv

593. The science which deals with the process of prevention of decay or spoilage of food thus allowing it to be stored for future use:

  A. Adulteration   B. Preservation

  C. Poisoning   D. None of the above

594. Microorganisms are different microscopic forms of both plant and animal life which includes:

  i. Moulds

  ii. Yeasts

  iii. Bacteria

  iv. Viruses

  A. i, ii, iii, iv   B. i, ii, iii

  C. i, ii   D. i, iv

595. Bacterias vary in their requirement of:

  i. Food

  ii. Moisture

  iii. pH

  iv. Temperature and oxygen

  A. i, ii, iii, iv

  B. i, ii, iii

  C. i, ii

  D. i, iv

596. Septic sore throat is caused by:

  A. Salmonella

  B. Staphylococci

  C. *Clostridium welchii*

  D. *Clostridium botulinum*

597. Staphylococci microorganisms are present in:

  A. Air   B. Water

  C. Boils   D. All of the above

598. The spores of _____ germinate in canned food.

  A. Staphylococci

  B. Botulinum

  C. Perfringens

  D. None of the above

599. The physical signs of the presence of *Clostridium botulinum* is/are:

  A. Gas presence

  B. Change in color

  C. Structural change

  D. All of the above

600. The physical appearance is like breads, it is:

  A. Clostridium

  B. Salmonella

  C. Staphylococci

  D. None of the above

601. Yeast fermentation produces chemical changes in which enzymes produced by the yeast cells converts:

  A. Alcohol into sugar

  B. Protein into amino acid

  C. Fats into fatty acids

  D. Sugar into alcohol

602. Bread, vinegar, beer and wine are produced with the help of:

  A. Mould   B. Bacteria

  C. Yeast   D. Enzymes

603. Aerobic and anaerobic bacteria may cause:

  A. Food spoilage

  B. Food poisoning

  C. Disease borne via food

  D. All of the above

604. The musty smell of spoiled grapes is due to:
A. Bacteria   B. Moulds
C. Yeast   D. Enzymes

605. Yeast produce, during their metabolism:
A. Undesirable chemical products
B. Pigments
C. Toxin
D. All of the above

606. Drying will not kill all bacteria. Upon hydrating certain dehydrated foods may lead to:
A. Better falvor
B. Better textile
C. Less cooking time
D. Spoilage

607. The life of every cell of plant or animal tissue depends upon the chemical reactions activated by:
A. Pigments   B. Oxygen
C. Enzymes   D. None of the above

608. Following are the types of pasteurization:
A. Holding process
B. High temperature short time
C. Flash process
D. All of the above

609. Which of the following factors should be examined in canning process?
i. Selection of food
ii. Sterilization of can
iii. Sealing of cans
iv. Storage
A. i, ii, iii, iv   B. i, ii, iii
C. i, ii   D. i, iv

610. Commercially sterile term is used for food:
A. Kept in refrigerator
B. Canned food without spoilage
C. Boiling of food
D. None of the above

611. Toxins produced by moulds growing on groundnuts and other agricultural products:
A. Mycotoxin
B. Enzymes
C. Aflatoxin
D. None of the above

612. Aerobic and anaerobic bacteria may cause:
A. Disease borne via food
B. Food poisoning
C. Food spoilage
D. All of the above

613. _____ is used as leavening in bread making. It gives the required flavor and sponginess to the bread.
A. Bacteria   B. Yeast
C. Mould   D. Enzymes

614. The life of every cell of plant or animal tissue depends upon the chemical reactions activated by:
A. Pigments
B. Oxygen
C. Enzymes
D. None of the above

615. The importance of food preservation in food industry is:
i. Shelf life and supply of food increases
ii. Seasonal foods are available throughout the year
iii. Variety of foods can be added
iv. Nutritional status is improved
A. i, ii, iii, iv
B. i, ii, iii
C. i, ii
D. None of these

616. Cooked food in refrigerator should be kept covered because:
A. Loss of moisture is prevented
B. Flavors do not mix
C. Keep bacteria away
D. All of the above

617. Canning method of preservation is applicable to:
   A. Fruit juices
   B. Syrups and sauces
   C. Fruit products
   D. All of the above

618. The vegetables are canned/bottled and sterilized by:
   A. Pressure cooker
   B. Boiling in hot water bath
   C. Washing with hot water
   D. None of the above

619. Mechanical device used for drying food is:
   A. Dehydrators   B. Roller dryers
   C. Spray dryers   D. All of the above

620. Temperature and humidity are controlled in mechanical drying for:
   A. Superior product
   B. Better color
   C. Correct texture
   D. All of the above

621. The use of roller drier or spray drier gives a product as:
   A. Crushed
   B. Ground
   C. Fine dry powder
   D. None of the above

622. Beverage powders like instant coffee and tea are spray dried:
   A. To make better powder
   B. Reconstitute better
   C. Tasteless bitter
   D. None of the above

623. Freeze dried foods are packed in the presence of:
   A. Oxygen
   B. Carbon dioxide
   C. Inert gas like nitrogen
   D. None of the above

624. Vegetables have to be given mild treatment called blanching that is above 80°C before they are frozen:
   A. To remove salt content
   B. To wash dirt away
   C. To prevent development of off-flavors
   D. None of the above

625. Certain substances retard or prevent the growth of microorganism. They are known as:
   A. Chemical
   B. Microorganism resistant
   C. Preservatives
   D. None of the above

626. Onion makes us cry when shedding. It is because in them are:
   A. Sulfur
   B. Acted upon by enzymes
   C. Produce volatile sulfur
   D. All of the above

627. Fruits stimulated to ripened by:
   A. Oxygen
   B. Carbon dioxide
   C. Ethylene gas
   D. None of the above

628. Beets and radish have _____ pigment.
   A. Anthocyanin   B. Flavones
   C. Flavonol   D. None of the above

629. Addition of baking soda for cooking causes:
   A. Increase water absorption
   B. Thiamine is lost
   C. Texture is affected
   D. All of the above

630. The quality of cow's milk depends on:
   A. Cow's feed
   B. Climate
   C. Texture is effected
   D. All of the above

631. When milk or cream is slowly churned fat molecules are formed and collect together on top, this is:

   A. Butter milk   B. Butter

   C. Cheese   D. Curd

632. The quality of cheese is effected by:

   i. Type of milk

   ii. The activity of curdling or coagulating milk

   iii. Moisture content

   iv. Cooking method

   A. i, ii, iii   B. ii, iii, iv

   C. iii, iv, i   D. i, ii, iii, iv

633. The function of chalazia in egg white is:

   A. Keep yolk in position

   B. Keep embryo in position

   C. Allows freedom of movement to both

   D. All of the above

634. The heat labile factor in egg white is called:

   A. Cholesterol   B. Heat resistant

   C. Avidin   D. None of the above

635. Egg is called acid producing food item because:

   A. Magnesium   B. Acid

   C. Sulfur   D. None of the above

636. When fat penetrates between the muscle fiber bundles of flesh meat this is called?

   A. Fat resistance   B. Marbling

   C. Heating   D. All of the above

637. Poultry includes:

   A. Chicken

   B. Ducks and geese

   C. Turkey and pigeons

   D. All of the above

638. Rigor mortis is:

   A. Loss of physical activity

   B. Cell chemical reaction

   C. Stiffening of the carcass

   D. None of the above

639. Rigor mortis affects by:

   i. Texture

   ii. Water holding capacity

   iii. Color

   iv. Flavor

   A. i, ii, iii, iv   B. i, ii, iii

   C. i, ii   D. i, iv

640. Mechanical method of tenderizing meat:

   i. Pounding

   ii. Cutting

   iii. Grinding

   iv. Needling or penning

   A. i, ii, iii, iv   B. i, ii, iii

   C. i, ii   D. i, iv

641. The flavor of fruit may be termed as:

   A. Taste

   B. Fragrant

   C. Sweet

   D. Any of these

642. Richest source of riboflavin is:

   A. Papaya

   B. Mango

   C. Woodapple (bael)

   D. Karonda

643. Tomato fruits for canning are harvested at:

   A. Mature green stage

   B. Red ripe stage

   C. Immature green stage

   D. Half ripe/pink stage

644. Which chemical is used for controlling sprouting of onions in storage?

   A. Maleic hydrazide

   B. Ethylene

   C. Methane

   D. Sulphur

645. Maximum tin content allowed in any canned food stuff is:

   A. 250 ppm   B. 500 ppm

   C. 600 ppm   D. 1000 ppm

646. Vegetables are subjected to drying after:
    A. Blanching
    B. Sulfuring
    C. Both of the above
    D. None of the above

647. Yellow colored vegetables and fruits are good source of:
    A. Vitamin D   B. Vitamin A
    C. Vitamin B   D. Vitamin C

648. Vegetable which is not blanched before drying is:
    A. Cauliflower   B. Spinach
    C. Onion   D. Tomato

649. The pink color of onion is due to presence of:
    A. Lycopene   B. Anthocyanin
    C. Quercitin   D. All of the above

650. Intake of iron and iodine gives protection against:
    A. Anemia and goiter
    B. Anemia and rickets
    C. Beriberi and goiter
    D. Osteoporosis and beriberi

651. Carotene in the body changes into vitamin A in the:
    A. Liver   B. Pancreas
    C. Gallbladder   D. Intestine

652. It is made in the body by the action of the Sun's rays on the fat under the skin:
    A. Vitamin D   B. Vitamin C
    C. Vitamin A   D. Vitamin B group

653. After absorption it reaches the thyroid gland and is oxidized:
    A. Fluorine   B. Iodine
    C. Zinc   D. Sulfur

654. It combines with iron to produce hemoglobin in the body:
    A. Copper   B. Zinc
    C. Sulfur   D. Sodium

655. Rice protein is of a better quality because of:
    A. Lysine   B. Tryptophan
    C. Threonine   D. None

656. Parboiled rice contains sufficient amount of:
    A. Nicotine   B. Thiamine
    C. Niacin   D. None of the above

657. Cereals are sources of:
    A. Calcium   B. Iron
    C. Cellulose   D. All of the above

658. Ragi is rich in:
    A. Calcium   B. Iron
    C. Cobalt   D. None of the above

659. Bajra is a good source of:
    A. Calcium   B. Iron
    C. Zinc   D. Cobalt

660. Phytate present in cereal _____ the absorption of iron.
    A. Increases   B. Decreases
    C. Neutralizes   D. None of the above

661. Suffering on account of substandard health is called:
    A. Mortality   B. Morbidity
    C. Morality   D. All of the above

662. Qualitative over nutrition may cause:
    A. Heart problem
    B. Hypertension
    C. Indigestion
    D. All of the above

663. Nutritional status is related to:
    A. Health   B. Vigor
    C. Achievement   D. All of the above

664. Any nutritive material of plant or animal origin which when taken into the human body meets the needs for growth maintenance tissue repair and work is:
    A. Nutrients   B. Food
    C. Medicine   D. None of the above

665. Soya bean is prescribed in the diet of diabetic patients because it is:
   A. High in protein
   B. Less in vitamin E
   C. Low in starch
   D. Good source of calcium, phosphorus, and iron.

666. When chlorophyll comes in contact with acids it changes to a dull olive green color called:
   A. Faded green
   B. Neutral green
   C. Pheophytin
   D. Soluble green

667. The pectin presents in fruit is useful for the production of:
   i. Pickels
   ii. Jams
   iii. Jelly
   iv. Crystallized fruits
   A. i, ii   B. iii, iv
   C. ii, iii   D. i, iv

668. Fleshy or pulpy in character often juicy and usually sweet with fragrant aromatic flavors:
   A. Vegetables   B. Fruits
   C. Cereals   D. None of the above

669. The flavor of fruit may be termed as:
   A. Taste   B. Fragrant
   C. Sweet   D. Any of these

670. When milk or cream is slowly churned fat molecules are formed and collect together on top, this is:
   A. Butter milk   B. Butter
   C. Cheese   D. Curdling

671. Cumin seeds have the property of:
   A. Stimulant
   B. Carminative
   C. Anticancer
   D. All of the above

672. It is ensured that the falvor of the food is retained because:
   A. Stimulates digestive juice secretions
   B. Aids effective digestive
   C. Helps assimilation of foods
   D. All of the above

673. When the flavor is drawn out:
   i. Aids digestion
   ii. Maximun digestion
   iii. Early spoilage
   iv. Less shelf life
   A. i, ii, iii, iv   B. i, ii, iii
   C. i, ii   D. i, iv

674. When bread is baked, potatoes are boiled and rice are cooked the heat of water effect starch granules:
   i. Swell up
   ii. Burst
   iii. Mix with water
   iv. Forms a paste
   A. i, ii, iii, iv   B. i, ii, iii
   C. i, ii   D. i, iv

675. When acid-rich fruits are cooked with the sugar changes into:
   i. Glucose
   ii. Fructose
   iii. Galactose
   iv. Sucrose
   A. i, ii, iii, iv   B. i, ii, iii
   C. i, ii   D. i, iv

676. To preserve murrabbas, jams and jellies the sugar:
   i. Sweetens
   ii. Binds moisture
   iii. Preserves
   iv. Digestive
   A. i, ii, iii, iv   B. i, ii, iii
   C. i, ii   D. i, iv

677. Compared to boiling and baking fried foods are:
   A. Attractive
   B. Tasty higher energy

C. Tasty

D. All of the above

678. Sodium, potassium and magnesium loss occurs by:

A. Blanching   B. Leaching

C. Soaking   D. None of the above

679. Fat is ready for use when:

  i. It is still

 ii. Blue flame arises

iii. Smells

 iv. Color changes

A. i, ii, iii, iv   B. i, ii, iii

C. i, ii   D. i, iv

680. To prevent vitamin C destruction from vegetables:

  i. Do not soak

 ii. Do not eat raw

iii. Do not store for long

 iv. Cook for less time

A. i, ii, iii, iv   B. i, ii, iii

C. i, ii   D. i, iv

681. Fish can be cooked by:

A. Dry heat boiling

B. Baking

C. Frying

D. All of the above

682. Poultry can be preserved and stored:

A. Canning

B. Dehydration and chilling

C. Freezing

D. All of the above

683. Steaming of vegetables is avoided because:

A. Slow method of cooking

B. Ascorbic acid loss

C. More fuel required

D. All of the above

684. Bottled milk exposed to strong sunlight lose of:

A. Protein   B. Fat

C. Carbohydrate   D. Riboflavin

685. Fruits cooked in metal contains form/do not:

A. Acid salts of metals

B. Alkaline salts

C. Neutralize

D. None of the above

686. Cooking in copper vessels and addition of soda cooking bad for:

  i. Vitamin B

 ii. Flavor

iii. Texture

 iv. Color

A. i, ii, iii, iv   B. i, ii, iii

C. i, ii   D. i, iv

687. Rancidity leads to the destruction of:

  i. Vitamin A

 ii. Vitamin E

iii. Vitamin B

 iv. Vitamin C

A. i, ii   B. iii, iv

C. i, iii   D. i, iv

688. While roasting food is turned around constantly because:

A. Heat is intense

B. Takes less time

C. Cooked from all sides

D. None of the above

689. Baking is slow method of cooking but food cooked is:

  i. Easily digestible

 ii. Not much loss of nutrients

iii. Tasty

 iv. Nutritive

A. i, ii, iii, iv   B. i, ii, iii

C. i, ii   D. i, iv

690. Peanut or popcorns are roasted in:

  i. Oven

 ii. Tandoor

iii. Hot sand

 iv. On flame

A. i, ii, iii, iv   B. i, ii, iv
C. ii, iii, iv   D. iii, iv, ii

691. The pan in stewing is covered for:
   i. Quick results
   ii. Save fuel
   iii. Minimum evaporation
   iv. Conserve nutrients and flavor
   A. i, ii, iii, iv   B. ii, iii, iv
   C. iii, iv   D. iv, i

692. In stewing food should be cut into small equal pieces for:
   A. Beauty
   B. Exposure to softening power of boiling water
   C. Makes bigger dish
   D. None of the above

693. The gravy of the stew should not have:
   i. A lot of thickness
   ii. Fat laden
   iii. To be thrown away
   iv. Spicy
   A. i, ii   B. ii, iii
   C. iii, iv   D. i, iv

694. Custards and pudding which are steamed are example of:
   A. Direct steaming
   B. Indirect steaming
   C. Pressure cooking
   D. None of the above

695. The best characteristic of pressure cooking is:
   A. Its sturdy body
   B. Time bound cooking
   C. High temperature reduces cooking time
   D. All of the above

696. Frying is suitable for:
   A. Invalids
   B. Foods that take short time to cook
   C. Taste
   D. None of the above

697. If the fat is over heated for frying food will:
   i. Cook well
   ii. Get burnt outside
   iii. Uncooked inside
   iv. Lose shape
   A. i, ii   B. ii, iii
   C. iii, iv   D. iv, i

698. The food is to be cooked can be dipped in besan egg or corn flour better in:
   A. Boiling   B. Shallow frying
   C. Deep frying   D. Baking

699. The role of salt in food preparation is:
   A. Seasoning
   B. Draws out water
   C. Binds water in solution
   D. All of the above

700. The roasting of cashew nut brings about:
   A. Browning
   B. Loss of thiamine
   C. Taste
   D. All of the above

701. Vitamin C is labile vitamin as:
   A. Water soluble
   B. Easily oxidized
   C. Effected by heat
   D. All of the above

702. Bottled milk exposed to strong sunlight lose of:
   A. Protein   B. Fat
   C. Carbohydrate   D. Riboflavin

703. Contamination with copper accelerates the rate of destruction of:
   A. Vitamin C   B. Vitamin A
   C. Vitamin B   D. Vitamin E

704. Cooking in copper vessels and addition of soda cooking is bad for:
   i. Vitamin B
   ii. Falvor

iii. Texture

iv. Color

A. i, ii, iii, iv   B. i, ii, iii

C. i, ii   D. i, iv

705. Rancidity leads to the destruction of:

   i. Vitamin A

   ii. Vitamin E

   iii. Vitamin B

   iv. Vitamin C

   A. i, ii   B. iii, iv

   C. i, iii   D. i, iv

706. Vitamin C and vitamin E, BHA and BHT, and sulfites are all:

   A. Falvor enhancer

   B. Antimicrobial agent

   C. Incidental food agent

   D. Antioxidants

707. Vitamin which is not found in fruits and vegetables is:

   A. Vitamin B_{12} B. Vitamin A

   C. Vitamin B_2 D. Vitamin C

708. Monosodium glutamate is used as:

   A. Source of amino acid

   B. Falvor enhancer

   C. Binder

   D. Moisture retainer

709. National pickle of India is:

   A. Lime pickle

   B. Mango pickle

   C. Cucumber pickle

   D. Carrot pickle

710. Egg shell is:

   A. Porous

   B. Non-porous

   C. None of theabove

   D. All of the above

711. Defects in fresh egg are:

   A. Meat spots   B. Cracks

   C. Bloom   D. All of the above

712. Which part of egg is richest in protein and fat:

   A. Egg white   B. Egg yolk

   C. Egg shell   D. Whole egg

713. Which part of egg contains cholesterol and thus restricted to cholesterol patient:

   A. Egg white   B. Egg yolk

   C. Egg shell   D. Whole egg

714. The bacterium capable of anaerobic nitrogen fixing is:

   A. Azotobacter   B. Bacillus

   C. Clostridium   D. Rhizopus

715. The term 'Microbiology' as study of living microorganisms, was coined by:

   A. AV Leewenhoek

   B. Robert Koch

   C. Louis Pasteur

   D. Edward Jenner

716. Which is an anti-hemorrhagic vitamin?

   A. Vitamin A   B. Vitamin K

   C. Vitamin E   D. Vitamin C

717. Which is known as vinegar bacteria?

   A. Lactobacillus

   B. Acetobacter

   C. Clostridium

   D. Bacillus

718. Which of the following has highest protein content?

   A. Oat   B. Ragi

   C. Wheat   D. Bajra

719. Which of the following has highest fat content?

   A. Rice   B. Bajra

   C. Maize   D. Oat

720. The MSNF means:

   A. Milk solid not fat

   B. Milk solid natural fat

   C. Milk solid non fat

   D. Milk standardized natural fat

721. Precursor of vitamin A is:
    A. Methionine
    B. β-carotene
    C. Tryptophan
    D. Ergosterol

722. Vitamin D increases the absorption of:
    A. Calcium and phosphorus
    B. Iron and calcium
    C. Sulfur and potassium
    D. Sodium and phosphorus

723. The major component of bacterial cell wall is a polymer called as:
    A. Xylan   B. Chitin
    C. Cellulose   D. Peptidoglycan

724. Which of the following is a reducing sugar?
    A. Starch   B. Lactose
    C. Fructose   D. Sucrose

725. Exhausting of cans is done to:
    A. Sterilize the cans
    B. Raise the sugar contents
    C. Remove the acid
    D. Expel the entrapped air in the contents

726. Calcium is used in human body for:
    A. Synthesis of bones
    B. Recovery of bicarbonate
    C. Utilization of sulfate
    D. Synthesis of amino acids

727. In the course of fermentation the quality of which of the nutrients is doubled:
    A. Thiamine   B. Riboflavin
    C. Niacin   D. All of the above

728. The advantages of germination are:
    i. Improved quality
    ii. Improved quantity
    iii. Digestibility
    iv. No extra cost
    A. i, ii, iii, iv   B. i, ii, iii
    C. i, ii   D. i, iv

729. The loss of vitamins during dehydration is affected by:
    A. Method of drying
    B. Stability of the vitamin
    C. Effect of air and heat
    D. All of the above

730. Alternatives to meat, fish and poultry as sources of protein are:
    A. Eggs   B. Shellfish
    C. Legumes   D. All of the above

731. Which of the following is not an intrinsic factor in food spoilage?
    A. pH
    B. Moisture content
    C. Available nutrients
    D. Temperature

732. There is an increased sensitivity to aflatoxins in individuals previously infected with:
    A. Hepatitis B   B. Measles
    C. Mumps   D. Chickenpox

733. Complex algal toxins, most of which are temperature stable, are known to cause peripheral neurological system effects, often in less than _____ after ingestion.
    A. One hour   B. Two hour
    C. Three hour   D. Four hour

734. Louis Pasteur established the modern era of food microbiology in 1857 when he showed that microorganisms cause _____ spoilage.
    A. Bear   B. Wine
    C. Juice   D. Milk

735. Several major brands of beer are _____ rather than pasteurized to better preserve the flavor and aroma of the original product.
    A. Centrifuged
    B. Filtered
    C. Heat treated
    D. All of the above

736. Which of the following terms describes organisms that thrive in the cold?

A. Mesophiles

B. Psychrophiles

C. Mesophiles

D. Thermophiles

737. Despite efforts to eliminate spoilage organisms during canning, sometimes canned foods are spoiled. This may be due to:

A. Spoilage before canning.

B. Under processing during canning

C. Leakage of contaminated water through can seams during cooling

D. All of the above

738. The effectiveness of many chemical preservatives depends primarily on the food:

A. Temperature   B. pH

C. Water content   D. Acidity

739. Sodium nitrite is responsible for:

A. Protecting against botulism

B. Reducing rate of spoilage

C. Maintenance of red color of meat

D. All of the above

740. Which of the following refers to the addition of microorganisms to the diet in order to provide health benefits beyond basic nutritive value?

A. Antibiotics   B. Adjuvants

C. Prebiotics   D. Probiotics

741. The main reservoir of *Staphylococcus aureus* is:

A. Human feces

B. Human nasal cavity

C. Blood cells

D. All of the above

742. Which one of the following is not an essential amino acid?

A. Lysine   B. Methionine

C. Alanine   D. Phenylalanine

743. Whiptail is a disorder which occur due to deficiency of:

A. Sulfur   B. Molybdenum

C. Zinc   D. Boron

744. Sulfur containing amino acid is:

A. Isoleucine   B. Valine

C. Cysteine   D. None of the above

745. National sugar institute is located at:

A. Varanasi   B. Kanpur

C. New Delhi   D. Lucknow

746. Biofertilizers are:

A. Green manures

B. Organic manures

C. Culture of microorganisms

D. None of the above

747. A nurse prepares an area of skin for injection by scrubbing it with an alcohol swab; this process is called:

A. Sanitation

B. Degerming

C. Sterilization

D. Disinfection

748. Which of the following terms includes the destruction of bacterial endospores?

A. Sterilization   B. Antisepsis

C. Sanitization   D. Pasteurization

749. All of the following microbes are killed by pasteurization *except*:

A. *Mycobacterium bovis*

B. *E. coli*

C. *Bacillus stearothermophilus*

D. *Brucella melitensis*

750. A particular machine passes milk through steam at a temperature of 140°C for one second and then cools it rapidly. This is an example of:

A. Ultrahigh-temperature pasteurization

B. Autoclaving

C. Pasteurization

D. Ultrahigh-temperature sterilization

751. All of the following microbial control methods are bacteriostatic *except*:

A. Lyophilization

B. Ionizing radiation

C. Desiccation

D. Refrigeration

752. All of the following are examples of ionizing radiation *except*:

A. Gamma rays

B. Ultraviolet light

C. X-rays

D. Electron beams

753. On a per weight basis which foodstuffs generate most energy:

A. Proteins   B. Fats

C. Carbohydrates   D. Fiber

754. Which hormone is secreted by the stomach when it is empty of food and stimulates appetite?

A. Ghrelin

B. Secretin

C. Leptin

D. Cholesystokinin

755. Why is protein a necessary component of the diet?

A. It provides essential fatty acids

B. Only half the amino acids found in proteins can be synthesized by the body

C. It is necessary for gluconeogenesis

D. It can be stored and used in fasting and starvation

756. Why do water soluble vitamins have to be taken in the diet more frequently than fat-soluble vitamins?

A. They are metabolized faster than the fat soluble vitamins

B. There are no extensive stores as any excess taken in the diet is excreted

C. Only small amounts are present in foodstuffs

D. They are destroyed by gastrointestinal flora

757. Which vitamin deficiency manifests itself as impaired wound healing, gastro-intestinal bleeding and sore and bleeding oral tissues?

A. Vitamin A   B. Folate

C. Vitamin C   D. Vitamin D

758. Which of the following statements about the digestion of proteins is correct?

A. Protein digestion begins in the small intestine

B. Protein digestion begins in the stomach

C. Protein digestion begins when the hydrochloric acid first hydrolyses the peptide bonds

D. Protein digestion begins when try-psinogen has been activated to trypsin by hydrochloric acid

759. Which of the following statements about food storage in the body is correct?

A. More glycogen is stored per unit mass in the muscles than in the liver

B. Glycogen storage in the liver is unli-mited

C. Fat is a more efficient form of fuel storage than glycogen

D. Proteins in muscle cells are a normal storage form of fuel

760. What is the function of chylomicrons?

A. They transport endogenously synthe-sized triacyl glycerols from the liver to the periphery

B. They are responsible for reverse cho-lesterol transport, i.e. from the peri-phery to the liver

C. They transport dietary fat from the intestine to the peripheral tissues

D. They transport cholesterol esters to peripheral tissues

761. Which of the following statements app-lies to the mucus that lines the gastro-intestinal tract?

A. Mucus is essentially composed of lipids

B. The only role of mucus is to help foods slide down the gastrointestinal tract

C. Mucus is secreted by goblet cells in the small intestine

D. Mucus is permeable to digestive enzymes

762. **Which of the following statements about circulating lipoproteins is correct?**

A. Chylomicrons release cholesterol to adipose tissues

B. VLDL release cholesterol to the liver

C. Chylomicrons contain mainly dietary triacylglycerols in their core

D. LDL contain mainly dietary triacylglycerols in their core

763. **Statins are drugs taken to lower blood cholesterol. What is their mode of action?**

A. They activate hormone sensitive lipase

B. They inhibit lipoprotein lipase

C. They inhibit HMG CoA reductase

D. They inhibit lecithin-cholesterol acyl transferase

764. **Which of the following statements about high density lipoprotein (HDL) is correct?**

A. HDL lipoproteins are only synthesized in the liver

B. HDL lipoproteins transport triacylglycerols to peripheral tissues

C. HDL lipoproteins pick up cholesterol and convert it to cholesterol ester

D. HDL lipoproteins cannot be endocytosed by the liver

765. **In the preparation of paneer from milk, the pH at which casein precipitate is?**

A. pH 6.5

B. pH 4.6

C. pH 7.5

D. pH 3.0

766. **The functionally active form of vitamin D is:**

A. Cholecalciferol

B. Ergocalciferol

C. Dehydrocholesterol

D. 1, 2, 5-Dihydroxycholecalciferol

767. **Factors responsible for browning of cut fruits are:**
   i. Oxygen
   ii. Phenolic compounds
   iii. Enzymes
   iv. Optimum pH
   Codes:

A. i, ii and iii   B. ii, iii and iv

C. ii, iii and iv   D. All of the above

768. **Germination enhances following nutrients:**
   i. Vitamin B
   ii. Vitamin C
   iii. Protein
   iv. Carbohydrates
   Codes:

A. i, ii, iii and iv are correct

B. i and ii are correct

C. iii and iv are correct

D. ii is correct

769. **Etiological factors for peptic ulcers are:**
   i. *Helicobacter pylori* infection
   ii. Eating habits
   iii. High cholesterol levels
   iv. Lack of exercise
   v. Hereditary factors
   Codes:

A. ii, iii and v

B. i, ii and v

C. i, iii and v

D. i, ii and iii

770. **Arrange the following steps in the preparation of peanut butter in correct sequence:**
   i. Grind the peanuts to a fine powder
   ii. Roast the peanuts and remove the skin
   iii. Beat mixture till creamy in texture
   iv. Add small amount of melted ghee and pinch of sugar and salt
   v. Transfer the contents to a sterilized jar
   Codes:

A. i, ii, iii, iv, v   B. ii, i, iv, iii, v

C. i, ii, iv, iii, v   D. ii, i, iii, iv, v

771. Arrange the following foods in decreasing order of vitamin B$_{12}$ content:
   i. Liver
   ii. Fish
   iii. Mutton
   iv. Milk
   Codes:
   A. i, ii, iii, iv   B. ii, iii, iv, i
   C. iii, i, ii, iv   D. iv, ii, i, iii

772. Arrange the following foods in decreasing order of vitamin B$_{12}$ content:
   i. Liver
   ii. Fish
   iii. Mutton
   iv. Milk
   Codes:
   A. i, ii, iii, iv
   B. ii, iii, iv, i
   C. iii, i, ii, iv
   D. iv, ii, i, iii

773. Match List-I with List-II:

List-I	List-II
A. Selenium	i. Garlic
B. Vitamin E	ii. Tomato
C. Flavonoids	iii. Sunflower seeds
D. Lycopene	iv. Seafoods
	v. Green leafy vegetables

   Codes:

	A	B	C	D
A.	iv	iii	i	ii
B.	iii	iv	ii	v
C.	ii	iii	v	i
D.	iv	v	ii	iii

774. Match the following diseases in List-I with their symptoms in List-II:

List-I	List-II
A. Diabetes	i. Heart burn
B. Atherosclerosis	ii. Proteinuria
C. Nephrotic syndrome	iii. Hypercholesterolemia
D. Cirrhosis	iv. Glycosuria
	v. Ascites

775. Match the items in List-I with items in List-II:

List-I	List-II
A. Dextrinization	i. Mayonaise
B. Gelatinization	ii. Peeled potatoes
C. Coagulation	iii. Kneading of dough
D. Emulsification	iv. Toasted bread
E. Enzymatic browning	v. Preparation of paneer
	vi. Preparation of white sauce

   Codes:

	A	B	C	D	E
A.	iv	iii	vi	i	v
B.	iii	v	vi	i	ii
C.	v	iv	iii	i	ii
D.	iv	vi	v	i	ii

   Codes:

	A	B	C	D
A.	iv	iii	ii	v
B.	iv	v	i	ii
C.	iii	ii	v	iv
D.	ii	iii	iv	i

776. Daily zinc requirement of an adult man is:
   A. 12 mg   B. 8 mg
   C. 350 mg   D. 600 mg

777. Infestation of which worm is responsible for the cause of anemia in rural population?
   A. Roundworm
   B. Hookworm
   C. Threadworm
   D. Tapeworm

778. Following is not a method of nutritional assessment using anthropometry:
   A. Skinfold thickness
   B. Waist circumference
   C. Blood pressure
   D. Midupper arm circumference

779. The hippocampus is found in:
    A. The circulatory system
    B. The human brain
    C. Fossils
    D. The preschool setting

780. Following are non-conventional novel foods developed for nutrition security:
    i. Leaf protein concentrate
    ii. Fermented foods
    iii. Spirulina
    iv. Textured soy protein
    v. Amylase rich food
    Codes:
    A. ii, v and i   B. i, ii, iii and iv
    C. iv, iii and ii   D. i, iii and iv

781. The requirements of following nutrients are increased during lactation:
    i. Protein
    ii. Vitamin A
    iii. Iron
    iv. Folic acid
    Codes:
    A. i, ii and iv   B. i, ii and iii
    C. i, iii and iv   D. All of the above

782. Which of the following methods of cooking food use moist heat?
    i. Poaching
    ii. Broiling
    iii. Sauteing
    iv. Stewing
    v. Braising
    Codes:
    A. i, ii, iv   B. i, iii, iv
    C. i, iv, v   D. i, ii, iii

783. Which of the following foods is rich source of omega-3 fatty acid?
    i. Walnuts
    ii. Fish
    iii. Butter
    iv. Egg

Codes:
    A. i and ii   B. ii and iv
    C. iii and iv   D. i and iii

784. Arrange the sequence of symptoms of vitamin A deficiency:
    i. Blindness
    ii. Xerosis of conjunctiva
    iii. Xerosis of cornea
    iv. Night blindness
    v. Bitot spot
    Codes:
    A. i, ii, iii, iv, v   B. iv, v, ii, iii, i
    C. ii, iii, i, v, iv   D. iv, ii, iii, v, i

785. HACCP is a preventive programme for hygienic control and food safety. Arrange the following steps of the HACCP system in their correct sequence:
    i. Identifying critical control points.
    ii. Monitoring each critical control point.
    iii. Developing criteria for control and prevention
    iv. Identification and assessment of hazards
    v. Taking immediate corrective action.
    Codes:
    A. iii, i, ii, v, iv
    B. iv, i, iii, ii, v
    C. iii, i, ii, iv, v
    D. iv, iii, i, ii, v

786. Arrange the following steps of bread making in the correct sequence:
    i. Keep dough for proofing
    ii. Add yeast and sugar to lukewarm water
    iii. Sieve refined flour and salt
    iv. Bake at 450°F in bread mould
    v. Knock back dough
    Codes:
    A. iii, i, ii, iv, v
    B. i, iii, iv, v, ii
    C. iii, ii, i, v, iv
    D. iii, v, ii, iv, i

787. Match the deficiency diseases from List-I with their symptoms in List-II:

List-I	List-II
A. Xerophthalmia	i. Glossitis
B. Beriberi	ii. Koilonychia
C. Ariboflavinosis	iii. Bow legs
D. Pellagra	iv. Keratomalacia
E. Anemia	v. Petechial hemorrhages
F. Rickets	vi. Diarrhea and dementia
G. Scurvy	vii. Neuropathy

Codes:

	A	B	C	D	E	F	G
A.	i	ii	iii	iv	v	vi	vii
B.	ii	iv	vii	v	iii	i	vi
C.	iv	v	vii	vi	iii	i	ii
D.	iv	vii	i	vi	ii	iii	v

788. Maillard reaction takes place in the following cooking procedure:

A. Prolonged cooking of milk with sugar
B. Prolonged cooking of milk with salt
C. Prolonged cooking of milk with vegetables
D. Prolonged cooking of milk with cereal

789. β-carotene in the body changes into retinol in:

A. Liver   B. Pancreas
C. Gallbladder   D. Intestine

790. Total parenteral nutrition involves:

A. Use of the large central vein to deliver life sustaining nourishment
B. Use of peripheral veins to deliver nourishment
C. Ingestion of food through the oral route
D. Use of a tube to deliver full fluid or commercial formulae

791. Following properties of egg are used in food preparation:

i. Emulsification
ii. Coagulation
iii. Tenderization
iv. Leavening

Codes:

A. i, ii and iii   B. ii, iii and iv
C. i, ii and iv   D. All of the above

792. Following nutrients play role in synthesis of hemoglobin:

i. Vitamin C
ii. Iron
iii. Vitamin B$_{12}$
iv. Protein

Codes:

A. ii and iii are correct
B. i and iv are correct
C. i, ii and iii are correct
D. All of the above are correct

793. Arrange the following steps in jelly preparation in the correct sequence:

i. Test the extract for pectin content
ii. Pour hot into sterilized jar
iii. Boil the fruit with citric acid and water until tender
iv. Wash and slice the fruit
v. Add sugar to extract and boil vigorously without stirring
vi. Strain the contents through muslin cloth to get clear extract
vii. Perform sheet test for readiness

Codes:

A. iv, iii, i, vii, vi, v, ii
B. iii, iv, vi, vii, i, v, ii
C. iv, v, vi, iii, i, vii, ii
D. iv, iii, vi, i, vi, vii, ii

794. Arrange the following vegetables in decreasing order of β-carotene:

i. Pumpkin
ii. Carrot
iii. Beet
iv. Green leafy vegetables

Codes:

A. i, ii, iii, iv   B. ii, iii, iv, i
C. iii, i, ii, iv   D. iv, ii, i, iii

795. Match the foods given in List-I with pigments given in List-II:

List-I	List-II
A. **Meat**	i. **Xanthophyll**
B. **Tomato**	ii. **Anthoxanthin**
C. **Brinjal**	iii. **Chlorophyll**
D. **Turnip**	iv. **Myoglobin**
E. **Corn**	v. **Anthocyanin**
	vi. **Lycopene**

Codes:

	A	B	C	D	E
A.	iv	iii	v	vi	i
B.	ii	i	v	vi	iii
C.	iv	vi	v	ii	i
D.	v	vi	iv	iii	i

796. Match the following processing methods in List-I with foods involved in List-II:

List-I	List-II
A. **Germination**	i. **Oils, butter, flours**
B. **Fermentation**	ii. **Dehydrated foods**
C. **Fortification**	iii. **Pulses, grains**
D. **Preservation**	iv. **Doughs and batters**

Codes:

	A	B	C	D
A.	iv	i	iii	ii
B.	iii	ii	i	iv
C.	ii	iii	i	iv
D.	iii	iv	i	ii

797. The fortificant used in iodized salt is:

A. Sodium iodide

B. Potassium iodate

C. Sodium iodate

D. Potassium iodide

798. Following is not a method of nutritional assessment using biochemical method:

A. Urinary iodine

B. Hemoglobin estimation

C. Serum retinol

D. Blood pressure

799. Electromyography is a method used for measuring:

A. Muscle fatigue

B. Electric phenomenon occurring in the muscle

C. Electric phenomenon occurring in the bones

D. Efficiency of tissues

800. Following food components have antioxidant effects:

i. **Sesame lignans**

ii. **Phenols**

iii. **Carotenoid**

iv. **Vitamin E**

v. **Vitamin D**

vi. **Vitamin C**

Codes:

A. iii, v, ii, vi   B. v, i, ii, iii

C. ii, iii, iv, vi   D. i, ii, iii, v

801. The following are the tests for measuring pectin concentration:

i. **Alcohol test**

ii. **Boiling point test**

iii. **Jelmeter test**

iv. **Sheet test**

Codes:

A. i and ii   B. ii and iv

C. i and iii   D. All of the above

802. Important functions of calcium are:

i. **Formation of bone**

ii. **Neuromuscular excitation**

iii. **Blood coagulation**

iv. **Membrane permeability**

v. **Maintain osmotic equilibrium**

Codes:

A. i and iv   B. i, ii, iii and iv

C. i, ii, iii and v   D. i, iii, iv and v

803. Fruits such as mangoes, papaya, peaches and apricots are rich source of:

i. **Antioxidants**

ii. **Carbohydrates**

iii. Soluble fiber

iv. Protein

Codes:

A. i, ii, iv   B. i, ii, iii

C. ii, iii, iv   D. None of the above

804. Mid-Day Meal (MDM) Programme for school children between 6 and 11 years of age involves the following:
   i. Monitors growth of the children
   ii. Provide 450 kcals and 8–12 g protein/day
   iii. Provide hot cooked meals
   iv. Provide timely immunization
   v. Improve school attendance
   Codes:

A. ii, iii and iv   B. ii, iii and v

C. i, ii and v   D. ii, iv and v

805. Common symptoms of Alzheimer's disease are:
   i. Disorientation
   ii. Joint pain
   iii. Anxiety and anger
   iv. Upper respiratory infections
   v. Memory loss
   Codes:

A. iv, i and v   B. ii, iv and i

C. iii, ii and v   D. i, iii and v

806. Oxidizing bleaching agents include:
   i. Sodium hypochlorite
   ii. Hydrogen peroxide
   iii. Ozone
   iv. Sodium bisulfate
   Codes:

A. ii, iii and iv are correct

B. i, ii and iii are correct

C. i, ii and iv are correct

D. i, iii and iv are correct

807. Arrange the steps used in planning of meals by using food exchange list:
   i. Use the food exchanges for planning menu
   ii. Distribute the above food exchanges between meals

iii. Estimate the amount of different food exchanges that provide required energy and protein (food exchange plan)

iv. Record personal data for determining RDA

Codes:

A. i, ii, iii, iv   B. iii, i, ii, iv

C. iv, ii, iii, i   D. iv, iii, ii, i

808. Arrange fruits in decreasing order as per their fiber content:
   i. Watermelon
   ii. banana
   iii. Papaya
   iv. Apple
   v. Sapota
   vi. Guava
   Codes:

A. iv, vi, v, i, ii, iii   B. vi, v, iv, iii, ii, i

C. ii, iv, iii, v, i, vi   D. ii, iv, i, vi, iii, v

809. Arrange in correct sequence the metabolic changes occurring in uncontrolled diabetic state:
   i. Dehydration
   ii. Glycosuria
   iii. Peripheral circulatory failure
   iv. Loss of water and electrolytes
   v. Anuria
   vi. Decrease renal blood flow
   vii. Coma and death
   Codes:

A. i, ii, iii, vi, v, iv, vii

B. ii, iv, i, iii, vi, v, vii

C. ii, i, iii, iv, vi, v, vii

D. ii, i, iv, iii, v, vi, vii

810. Match the disease condition given in List-I with the nutrient to be restricted given in List-II:

List-I	List-II
A. Celiac	i. Fiber
B. Typhoid	ii. Sodium
C. Renal failure	iii. Gluten
D. Atherosclerosis	iv. Fat

E. Liver   v. **Saturated fatty acids**

F. **Hypertension**   vi. **Medium chain triglycerides**

vii. **Protein**

Codes:

	A	B	C	D	E	F
A.	ii	vi	iv	i	v	iii
B.	iv	vii	i	v	vi	ii
C.	iii	i	vii	v	iv	ii
D.	iii	vii	ii	iv	vi	i

811. **Match the microorganism given in List-I with the food-borne disease condition in List-II:**

List-I

A. **Salmonella**

B. **Shigella**

C. **Clostridium**

D. **Protozoa**

E. **Virus**

List-II

i. **Dysentery**

ii. **Amoebic dysentery**

iii. **Tuberculosis**

iv. **Hepatitis**

v. **Enteric fever**

vi. **Botulism**

Codes:

	A	B	C	D	E
A.	ii	v	i	vi	iii
B.	v	iii	ii	vi	iv
C.	v	i	vi	ii	iv
D.	i	v	vi	ii	iii

812. **Visual diagrams that provide a variety of food recommendations to help a person create a well-balanced diet:**

A. Food guidance systems

B. Dietary reference intakes

C. Dietary guidelines for Americans

D. Recommended dietary allowances

813. **A nutrient that can help lower blood pressure is:**

A. Potassium

B. Fat

C. Sodium

D. Protein

814. **It is recommended that we consume mostly unsaturated fats, such as those found in:**

A. Hydrogenated fat

B. Vegetable oil

C. Whole milk

D. Refined oil

815. **Regular physical activity helps a person to:**

A. Increase body weight

B. Decrease the amount of sleep required

C. Decrease the risk of chronic diseases

D. Increase intake of dietary fats

816. **The amount of nutrients a food contains in relationship to the number of calories it contains is:**

A. Caloric density   B. Personalization

C. Proportionality   D. Nutrient density

817. **Foods high in added sugars and saturated fats are:**

A. Less nutrient dense

B. High in fiber

C. Not allowed in the diet

D. Low in caloric content

818. **Whole grains include:**

A. White rice   B. Oats

C. Potato   D. Wheat bread

819. **One ounce equivalent (1 oz. eq) from the meat and beans group includes:**

A. Two (2) eggs

B. One-quarter (1/4) cup of cooked dry beans

C. Two (2) tablespoons of peanut butter

D. One (1) ounce of nuts

820. **The nutrition facts panel of the food label must provide:**

A. Health claims

B. Trans fat content

C. Recipes for using the food product

D. Exchange list

821. **Salmon and sardines contain a compound that may help to lower:**

    A. Heart disease   B. Blood sugar

    C. Blood pressure   D. Blood cholesterol

822. **There are no daily values (DV) listed for trans fats and sugar because:**

    A. There is no need to control the intake of these items

    B. There is not enough information available to set reference values for them

    C. They only appear in small quantities

    D. They are natural substances found in food

823. **A claim on the label that describes a relationship between a food and a disease is called a:**

    A. Nutrient claim

    B. Approved claim

    C. Structure/function claim

    D. Health claim

824. **Carbohydrates, lipids, and proteins all contain carbon, hydrogen, and oxygen. Which one also contains nitrogen?**

    A. Carbohydrates   B. Lipids

    C. Proteins   D. None of the above

825. **A function of carbohydrates in the diet is to:**

    A. Enable chemical reactions

    B. Promote growth and repair of tissues

    C. Supply energy

    D. Maintain water balance

826. **Good sources of carbohydrate are:**

    A. Fats, oils, butter, and margarine

    B. Fish, eggs, beef, pork, and poultry

    C. Cereals, fruits, vegetables, and milk

    D. Green leafy vegetables, seafood, and water

827. **Functions of lipids in the diet are to:**

    A. Provide fats essential for body function

    B. Transport water-soluble vitamins

    C. Promote growth and repair of tissue

    D. Maintain fluid balance

828. **Lipids are supplied in large quantities in the diet by:**

    A. Fats, oils, meats, and nuts

    B. Cereals, fruits, vegetables, and breads

    C. Deep green and orange vegetables

    D. Green pepper, broccoli, cantaloupe, and citrus fruits

829. **A function of protein is to:**

    A. Provide essential fatty acids

    B. Promote growth and repair of the body

    C. Participate in nervous system functioning

    D. Medium for temperature regulation

830. **Good sources of protein in the diet are:**

    A. Fats, oils, butter, and margarine

    B. Green pepper, cantaloupe, citrus fruits, and broccoli

    C. Meats, fish, legumes, nuts, dairy products, and eggs

    D. Deep green and orange vegetables and citrus fruits

831. **Essential nutrients:**

    A. Are made by the body

    B. Generally must be supplied by food

    C. Include alcohol

    D. All enzymes

832. **A kilocalorie (kcal) is a:**

    A. Measure of fat weight

    B. Unit for expressing energy content in food

    C. Scientific instrument

    D. Term used to describe the amount of sugar and fat in a food

833. **The building blocks of proteins are:**

    A. Amino acids

    B. Fatty acids

    C. Glucose units

    D. Coenzymes

834. The average amount of fat in the human body:
    A. Is almost the same as the amount of fat in broccoli and meat
    B. Represents most of the body weight for males and females
    C. Is typically greater in women than men
    D. Is equal to the weight of the muscle tissue

835. Nutrients that supply energy are:
    A. Fats and vitamins
    B. Minerals and water
    C. Minerals and vitamins
    D. Fats and carbohydrates

836. Adequate, regular physical activity:
    A. Prevents some adult bone loss
    B. Can actually replace the need for a healthy diet
    C. Requires that adults must take supplements since they cannot get all the nutrients they need from food when they are exercising regularly
    D. Must be done for at least two hours seven days a week

837. The benefits of regular, moderate physical activity include:
    A. Reduced risk for developing obesity
    B. Fewer infections
    C. Fewer injuries
    D. All of the above

838. The form of energy used by cells is called:
    A. Adenosine diphosphate
    B. Glucose
    C. Phosphocreatine
    D. Adenosine triphosphate

839. When glucose is broken down in an environment where oxygen supply is limited, a 3-carbon component known as _____ accumulates in the muscle.
    A. Glycogen　　　　B. Lactate
    C. Nitrogen　　　　D. Creatinine

840. When there is plenty of oxygen available in the muscles, the condition is referred to as being:
    A. Anaerobic　　　　B. Oxygenated
    C. Aerobic　　　　　D. Ventilated

841. What is the major disadvantage of accumulating lactate in the muscles?
    A. Fatigue
    B. Muscle damage
    C. Nausea
    D. None; it is an advantage

842. The site of greatest energy production in a muscle cell is the:
    A. Cytoplasm　　　　B. Mitochondria
    C. Ribosomes　　　　D. Nucleus

843. Athletes may take carnitine pills in order to _____. However, this is of no demonstrable value.
    A. Provide glycogen stores
    B. Build muscles
    C. Burn fat faster
    D. Increase foot speed

844. Athletes may take carnitine pills in order to _____. However, this is of no demonstrable value.
    A. Build muscles
    B. Increase foot speed
    C. Burn fat faster
    D. Provide glycogen stores

845. What source of energy is mainly used in light, aerobic activity?
    A. Carbohydrate　　　B. Fat
    C. Protein　　　　　D. All of the above

846. Which of the foods below constitutes the best choice when one attempts carbohydrate loading before endurance events?
    A. Potato chips
    B. French fries
    C. All bran (high fiber) cereal
    D. Rice

847. It is a good idea, especially for adult women athletes, to have blood hemoglobin regularly checked to detect for a possible deficiency of what mineral?

    A. Calcium   B. Potassium
    C. Copper   D. Iron

848. A light meal is best eaten _____ before participating in a sporting event.

    A. 1 hour
    B. Immediately before to give a boost of energy
    C. 2 to 4 hours
    D. 8–10 hours

849. Which of the answers below describes the benefit of a "sports" drink?

    A. Provides water to hydrate
    B. Provides electrolytes to enhance water absorption in the intestine and to maintain blood volume
    C. Supplies carbohydrate to provide energy
    D. All of the above

850. Minerals constitute about _____ % of the total body weight.

    A. 2   B. 4
    C. 6   D. 8

851. Each gram of dietary protein provides about 4 calories, a gram of fat provides about _____ calories.

    A. 5   B. 7
    C. 9   D. 11

852. The vitamin essential to the absorption and utilization of calcium and phosphorus is vitamin _____.

    A. C   B. E
    C. A   D. D

853. The vitamin essential for the formation of photopigments of the retina is vitamin _____.

    A. C   B. E
    C. A   D. B

854. The term metabolism refers to:

    A. Anabolic reactions
    B. Catabolic reactions
    C. Oxidation
    D. All chemical reactions of the body.

855. The breakdown of complex organic molecules into smaller ones is known as:

    A. Anabolism   B. Catabolism
    C. Metabolism   D. Oxidation

856. A chemical reaction that requires energy is:

    A. Anabolism   B. Catabolism
    C. Metabolism   D. Oxidation

857. Each gram of a carbohydrate produces about:

    A. 2.0 kilocalories
    B. 4.0 kilocalories
    C. 6.0 kilocalories
    D. 8.0 kilocalories

858. Glucose is stored in the liver and muscles as:

    A. Starch   B. Cellulose
    C. Fat   D. Glycogen

859. The rate of glucose transport across cell membranes is greatly increased by:

    A. Insulin   B. Glucagon
    C. Thyroxin   D. Calcium

860. Glycogen breakdown occurs when:

    A. Blood levels of glucose drop
    B. Glucagon is released
    C. Blood levels of glucose are high
    D. Both A and B

861. The formation of glucose from proteins and fats is called:

    A. Glycogenolysis   B. Lipolysis
    C. Glycogenesis   D. Gluconeogenesis

862. Ketone bodies are the result of catabolism of:

    A. Glycerol   B. Fatty acids
    C. Amino acids   D. Glycogen

863. Before entering the Krebs cycle, fatty acids are converted into molecules of:

A. Glucose

B. Glyceraldehyde-3 phosphate

C. Pyruvic acid

D. Acetyl CoA

864. Excess carbohydrates are synthesized into:

A. Amino acids   B. Proteins

C. Triglycerides   D. Ketone bodies

865. During digestion, proteins are broken down into molecules of:

A. Glucose   B. Fatty acids

C. Glycerol   D. Amino acids

866. Protein synthesis occurs in:

A. Ribosomes   B. Mitochondria

C. Lysosomes   D. Golgi complexes

867. Which of the following vitamins can be made by the body?

A. Vitamins C and B   B. Vitamins D and K

C. Vitamins E and B   D. Vitamins K and C

868. Which of the following vitamins is water-soluble?

A. Vitamin B   B. Vitamin A

C. Vitamin D   D. Vitamin E

869. Which of the following factors affect the metabolic rate?

A. Exercise   B. Age

C. Gender   D. All of the above

870. Which of the following hormones regulates the basal state of metabolism?

A. Vasopressin   B. Thyroxin

C. Insulin   D. Estrogen

871. The transfer of heat from a warmer object to a cooler one without physical contact is called:

A. Conduction   B. Evaporation

C. Convection   D. Radiation

872. The thermostat of the human body is located in the:

A. Thalamus

B. Hypothalamus

C. Cortex

D. Medulla oblongata

873. All of the following results in an increase of body temperature *except*:

A. Vasoconstriction

B. Vasodilation

C. Epinephrine release

D. Release of thyroid hormones

874. In degrees of celsius normal body temperature is near:

A. 35   B. 37

C. 39   D. 40

875. Sympathetic stimulation:

A. Increases cellular metabolism

B. Decreases cellular metabolism

C. Has no effect on cellular metabolism

D. Decreases body temperature

876. Which of the following compounds transport dietary lipids to adipose tissue for storage?

A. Chylomicrons

B. Low density lipoproteins

C. High density lipoproteins

D. Peripheral proteins

877. Which of the following hormone(s) is the main regulators of the basal metabolic rate?

A. Human growth hormone

B. Testosterone

C. Thyroid hormones

D. Insulin

878. Basal metabolic rate:

A. Reflects the rate nutrients are metabolized when one is exercising

B. Reflects nitrogen consumption

C. Remains constant throughout the day

D. None of the above are true of basal metabolism

879. The process of deamination refers to:

A. Someone with an abnormally low basal metabolic rate

B. The removal of a nitrogen from an amino acid

C. The anabolism of amino acids into proteins

D. The increase in basal metabolic rate that comes from an excess of proteins

880. Energy derived from nutrients is measured in:

A. Ergs   B. Kilocalories

C. Newtons   D. None of the above

881. Which of the following is not true about minerals?

A. They are inorganic

B. They are needed in small quantities

C. Levels are controlled by hormones

D. They can be synthesized by the body

882. Which of the following is examples of poor nutrition?

A. Iodine deficiency

B. Obesity

C. Kwashiorkor

D. All are examples of poor nutrition

883. Which of the following does not provide most of the energy for high intensity exercise?

A. Anaerobic glycolysis

B. Lipid catabolism

C. ATP

D. Creatine phosphate

884. A type of under nutrition resulting from an inadequate diet in protein and calories is called:

A. Kwashiorkor   B. Marasmus

C. Anemia   D. Obesity

885. What fate do food molecules absorbed by the GI tract have?

A. Supply energy

B. Synthesis of more complex molecules

C. Anabolism or catabolism

D. All of the above

886. "Good" cholesterol is:

A. LDL

B. VLDL

C. Chylomicrons

D. HDL

887. All of the following are correct about pasteurization _except_:

A. It is important in the dairy and juice industry

B. It does not alter the taste of the food

C. That it was developed in 1864 by Louis Pasteur

D. It eliminates all microbes

888. Which is the important flavor enhancer?

A. Vitamin A

B. Vitamin C

C. Monosodium glutamate

D. Aspartame

889. Since nitrosamines have been found to be carcinogenic in animals, the FDA requires that all foods with nitrites must also contain:

A. EDTA (ethylenediaminetetra-acetic acid)

B. Calcium propionate

C. Sulphites

D. Antioxidants

890. Which of the following additives can cause adverse asthmatic reactions in sensitive people?

A. Butylated hydroxytoluene (BHT)

B. Propyll gallate

C. Nitrates

D. Sulphites

891. Which of the following is the toxin found in green potatoes?

A. Botulism toxin   B. Solanine

C. Aflatoxin   D. Mycotoxin

892. Which of the following microbes would be most likely found in improperly canned foods?

A. *Campylobacter jejuni*

B. Salmonella

C. *Escherichia coli*

D. *Clostridium botulinum*

893. "Juice boxes" would be an example of the preservation technique of:

A. Irradiation   B. Freeze-drying

C. Sugaring   D. Aseptic packaging

894. What is the preferred source of energy for the brain?

A. Glucose   B. Maltose

C. Fructose   D. Maltose

895. What is high-fructose corn syrup?

A. A sugar created by heating sucrose syrup and adding chloride molecules

B. A man-made artificial sweetener with zero kilocalories

C. A common sugar alcohol

D. A nutritive sweetener made from corn syrup that is frequently used by the soda industry

896. Which of the following is table sugar?

A. Glucose   B. Fructose

C. Galactose   D. Sucrose

897. Where does sucrose come from?

A. Corn syrup produced from corn

B. Sugarcane or sugar beets

C. Maple syrup and honey

D. A soy byproduct

898. Fibers originate from which category of food?

A. Dairy   B. Seafoods

C. Plants   D. Animal foods

899. Which enzyme is lacking among people who find it uncomfortable to drink large volumes of milk?

A. Lactase   B. Maltase

C. Sucrase   D. Amylase

900. Ketoacidosis is frequently found among which category of patients?

A. Hypertension

B. Heartburn

C. Alzheimer's disease

D. Diabetes

901. Which nutrient provides amino acids:

A. Minerals   B. Carbohydrates

C. Proteins   D. Vitamins

902. Iodine, potassium, sodium, zinc, and calcium are all:

A. Vitamins   B. Carbohydrates

C. Proteins   D. Minerals

903. Which nutrient is a concentrated form of energy?

A. Fats   B. Carbohydrates

C. Proteins   D. Vitamins

904. The formula for body mass indexing is:

A. Height divided by weight

B. Weight divided by height

C. Weight divided by height squared

D. Height divided by weight squared

905. There are six classes of nutrients that humans need in order to function properly. Which of the following is not a class of nutrients?

A. Water   B. Fats

C. Meats   D. Vitamins

906. Vitamin C was first discovered:

A. In the 19th century, when a British doctor observed that his sick son, who could only stomach oranges, seemed to recover more quickly than his twin brother (also sick) who would only eat pasta

B. In 1800, in a British lab, by several scientists who were studying the pigmentation of the orange

C. In 1743, when a British navy surgeon, faced with the prospect of his entire crew succumbing to scurvy, discovered that citrus fruits could alleviate the symptoms of scurvy

D. In the latter half of the 19th century, during a botched game of horseshoes. The horseshoe landed on a nearby servant who happened to be eating a citrus fruit (a fruit unknown in the new colonies but had just been sent over by the servant's mother). Unfortunately, the servant died, but a nearby scientist became intrigued by this new fruit. The vitamin found to be present in the fruit was named C in honor of the shape of the horseshoe.

907. Saturated fats have been shown to increase blood cholesterol levels, a risk factor in heart disease. Which of the following, per serving, is highest in saturated fat?

A. Butter   B. Olive oil

C. Fish oil   D. None of the above

908. Which of the following is one of the functions of protein?

A. It regulates biochemical reactions

B. It is essential for the growth and repair of all body tissues

C. It insulates the body, protecting organs and nerve pathways

D. It breaks down into glucose, thereby providing fuel for the body

909. Which of the following is not a good source of vitamin C?

A. Potatoes   B. Strawberries

C. Chickpeas   D. Grapefruit

910. At 9 calories per gram, which is the most concentrated source of food energy?

A. Proteins

B. Carbohydrates

C. Vitamins

D. Fats

911. Which of the following is not a function of fiber?

A. It supplies the body with energy

B. It regulates bowel functions

C. It reduces the risk of intestinal problems

D. It promotes feelings of fullness

912. The mineral iron:

A. If ingested in excess, will give the skin a greenish hue

B. Is only found in red meat and liver

C. Is an essential part of hemoglobin—the substance which carries oxygen in the blood

D. When taken with protein, forms a complex carbohydrate

913. Which vitamin is known to help construct DNA as well as prevent birth defects?

A. Magnesium

B. Folic acid

C. Potassium

D. Riboflavin

914. Water is most important nutrient for body. Which of the following is not a function of water?

A. It transports nutrients

B. It lubricates and cushions organs

C. It maintains your body temperature

D. It fuels the body

915. Omega-3 fatty acids are very important for normal brain development, communication, and vision. Omega-3 fatty acids are:

A. Essential fatty acids that your body cannot synthesize from other nutrients

B. Found in high concentrations in genetically engineered carrots. This process increases the concentration of unsaturated fat in the carrots.

C. Essential to your body's ability to store glycogen

D. Found in foods such as breads, grains, cereals, and pasta

916. According to the majority of current research, which of the following is a beneficial effect of the trace mineral chromium?

A. It builds muscle tissue

B. It enhances athletic performance

C. By enhancing the activity of insulin, chromium helps the body to maintain glucose homeostasis

D. It retards cancer cell growth and lowers the risk of colon cancer

917. Which vitamin can be manufactured in the body from non-dietary sources?

A. Vitamin B_{12} B. Vitamin D

C. Vitamin E   D. Vitamin A

918. A protein is composed of _____, which help to build _____.

A. Amino acids/muscle mass

B. Simple sugars/complex carbohydrates

C. Fatty acid molecules/bones

D. Glucose molecules/carbohydrates

919. Water can contain varying amounts of minerals. If it contains more _____, it is termed "hard" and if it contains more _____, it is termed "soft".

A. Sodium/calcium

B. Potassium/magnesium

C. Magnesium/calcium and potassium

D. Calcium and magnesium/sodium

920. Foods with "empty calories" are those that:

A. Have less than 0.5 grams of fat

B. Have very little, if any, nutritional value

C. Are packed with vitamins but do not offer much in terms of energy

D. Contain less than 150 calories per serving

921. Which of the following two vitamins are known to be antioxidants (i.e. fight against free radicals)?

A. Vitamins C and E

B. Vitamins B_6 and B_{12}

C. Vitamins A and C

D. Vitamins E and K

922. The three main groups of carbohydrates are:

A. Monosaccharides

B. Disaccharides

C. Polysaccharides

D. All of the above

923. The condition which occurs due to excess dose of vitamin is:

A. Hypertension

B. Hypovitaminosis

C. Hypervitaminosis

D. Hyperglycemia

924. The amount of water present in butter is:

A. 20%   B. 16%

C. 18%   D. None of the above

925. Wheat germ is a good source of:

A. Vitamin A

B. Vitamin B complex and E

C. Vitamin C

D. All of the above

926. The percentage of fat present in heavy cream:

A. 30–40%   B. 60–80%

C. 35–50%   D. 40–60%

927. Butter, margarine and cooking oil are:

A. Visible fats   B. Invisible fats

C. Both A and B   D. None of the above

928. Fibrous form of carbohydrates that cannot be digested:

A. Cellulose   B. Saccharin

C. Pectin   D. All of the above

929. **Which fruit is most suitable for making jelly:**
    A. Mango   B. Papaya
    C. Lichee   D. Guava

930. **Pungency of raddish is due to presence of:**
    A. Solanine   B. Capsaicin
    C. Isothiocyanate D. Calcium acetate

931. **Glycogen is stored in:**
    A. Pancreas   B. Liver
    C. Teeth   D. Stomach

932. **The pungency of mustard oil is due to presence of which chemical compounds?**
    A. Phenols   B. Amino acid
    C. Glucosilates   D. Solanine

933. **Operation flood is associated with:**
    A. Soil erosion
    B. Flood control
    C. Increase in milk production
    D. Increase in oil production

934. **The digestion of fats mainly occur in the:**
    A. Large intestine B. Small intestine
    C. Liver   D. Pancreas

935. **Which of the following is not a micronutrient?**
    A. Copper   B. Boron
    C. Sulfur   D. Manganese

936. **Which of the following is a micronutrient?**
    A. Magnesium   B. Zinc
    C. Phosphorus   D. Potassium

937. **An inadequate supply of essential nutrients in the diet may result in:**
    A. Overnutrition B. Malnutrition
    C. Good nutrition D. All of the above

938. **Who is the father of white revolution?**
    A. Indira Gandhi
    B. Bill Gates

    C. Dr V Kurein
    D. Pt Jawaharlal Nehru

939. **Complete proteins contain all the essential:**
    A. Fatty acids   B. Amino acids
    C. Minerals   D. Vitamins

940. **The red color of blood is due to presence of:**
    A. Hemoglobin   B. Carotene
    C. Heparin   D. None of the above

941. **Nitrogen-containing chemical compounds of which protein is composed are:**
    A. Carbohydrates B. Amino acids
    C. Fatty acids   D. All of the above

942. **Iron is known to be necessary component of:**
    A. Hemoglobin   B. Bile juice
    C. Lymph   D. All of the above

943. **Iodine is essential to health:**
    A. Effects the rate of metabolism
    B. Deficiency causes goiter
    C. Both a and b
    D. None of the above

944. **How many amino acids are necessary for the body?**
    A. 21   B. 20
    C. 28   D. 25

945. **The body makes protein out of:**
    A. Carbohydrates B. Fatty acids
    C. Amino acids   D. Sugar

946. **Which nutrient is used as immediate fuel and converted to glucose?**
    A. Carbohydrates B. Proteins
    C. Vitamins   D. Minerals

947. **After the body's carbohydrate reserves are depleted, what does the body burn?**
    A. Proteins
    B. Vitamins and minerals

C. Lipids

D. All of the above

948. Which of the following helps treat and prevent constipation, hemorrhoids, diverticular disease and irritable bowel syndrome?

A. Fiber   B. Fats

C. Salt   D. None of the above

949. What are the important functions of lipids?

A. To insulate the body

B. To protect organs of body

C. To provide energy

D. All of the above

950. An excess of what can lead to increased levels of triglycerides and cholesterol in the blood and an increased risk of heart and artery disease?

A. Proteins   B. Fats

C. Fiber   D. Carbohydrates

951. An increased intake of soluble fiber, a decrease in the dietary intake of saturated fats and exercise result in:

A. Reduced vitamin contents

B. Reduced cholesterol contents

C. Reduced carbohydrates contents

D. Reduced minerals contents

952. What builds healthy bones and teeth, aids in blood clotting and helps nerves and muscles function?

A. Magnesium   B. Calcium

C. Selenium   D. Zinc

953. Which mineral works with vitamin E to aid metabolism, growth and fertility?

A. Selenium   B. Zinc

C. Copper   D. Magnesium

954. The color of beetroot is due to presence of:

A. Carotene   B. Capsaicin

C. Betanin   D. Anthocyanin

955. Which vitamin is found in yellow and orange fruits and vegetables?

A. Vitamin D   B. Vitamin B_1

C. Vitamin A   D. Vitamin C

956. What maintains fluid and acid–base balance and its main dietary source is salt?

A. Copper   B. Zinc

C. Selenium   D. Sodium

957. What represents an important dietary change for the elderly patient?

A. Increase fats and sugar

B. Increase high fiber foods and water

C. Both A and B

D. None of the above

958. What are the important signs and symptoms of anorexia nervosa?

A. Cessation of menstruation

B. Denial of hunger

C. Both a and b

D. None of the above

959. The term protein was given by:

A. Venda   B. Watson

C. Rose   D. Mulder

960. Egg yolk is a good source of:

A. Fat   B. Protein

C. Both   D. None of the above

961. Fishy odor in rotten egg is due to:

A. Bacteria (*E. coli*) B. Virus

C. Fungi   D. None of the above

962. Grading of egg is done on the basis of:

A. Shape and size of egg

B. Air cell size

C. Blood and meat spot

D. All of the above

963. The outer protective covering of shell is made up of:

A. Magnesium carbonate

B. Calcium carbonate ($CaCO_3$)

   C. Hydrogen oxide

   D. All of the above

964. Grading of egg is done by:

   A. Candler   B. Brodder

   C. Incubator   D. Hatcher

965. The most common cause of food-borne illness is the presence of what in foods:

   A. Bacteria

   B. Chemical preservatives

   C. Viruses

   D. Molds

966. Pasteurization involves the:

   A. Exposure of food to heat to inactivate enzymes that cause undesirable effects in foods during storage

   B. Exposure of food to high temperatures for short periods to destroy harmful microorganisms

   C. Fortifications of foods with vitamin A and vitamin D

   D. Use of irradiation to destroy certain pathogens in foods

967. Those at greatest risk for food-borne illness include:

   A. Pregnant woman

   B. Infants and children

   C. Immunosuppressed children

   D. All of the above

968. Ancient methods of food preservation include:

   A. Pasteurizing and sterilizing

   B. Canning, blanching, and irradiating

   C. Freezing and boiling

   D. Drying, smoking, and fermenting

969. A biological method of food preservation is:

   A. Freezing

   B. Drying

   C. Fermenting

   D. Adding salt

970. The organisms used in the process of fermentation:

   A. Metabolize all the oxygen in food

   B. Produce water in the food

   C. Utilize all the nutrients in the food

   D. Produce products such as acids, that inhibit the growth of other microorganisms

971. Food can be kept for long periods of time by adding salt or sugar because these substances:

   A. Make the food too acidic for spoilage to occur

   B. Bind to water, thereby making it unavailable to the microorganisms

   C. Effectively kills microorganisms

   D. Dissolve the cell walls in plant foods

972. Bacteria that can grow in the absence of oxygen are called:

   A. Anaerobes   B. Aerobes

   C. Molds   D. Yeasts

973. A danger of using home-canned food if the processing has been inadequate is:

   A. Cancer

   B. Botulism

   C. Excessive nutrient loss

   D. Excessive tin in the juice

974. _____ creates free radicals in food, which can destroy cell membranes and attack DNA and proteins, thus preventing microorganism growth.

   A. Pasteurization   B. Irradiation

   C. Reduction   D. All of the above

975. Milk that can remain on supermarket shelves, free of microbial growth, for many years has been processed by which of the following methods?

   A. Use of humectants

   B. Use of antibiotics in animal feed

   C. Sequestrants

   D. Aseptic processing

976. It is unwise to thaw meats or poultry:

A. In a microwave oven

B. In the refrigerator

C. Under cool running water

D. At room temperature

977. Keeping food above 140°F (60°C):

A. Increases microbial growth

B. Slows chemical deterioration

C. Stops chemical reactions

D. Reduces the growth of pathogens

978. Salmonella bacteria are usually spread via:

A. Raw meats, poultry, and eggs

B. Pickled vegetables

C. Home canned vegetables

D. Raw vegetables

979. The food-borne illness organism often associated with small cuts and boils is:

A. Listeria

B. Staphylococcus

C. C. botulinum

D. Salmonella

980. Food additives may be used to:

A. Destroy nutrients

B. Disguise faulty products

C. Deceive customers

D. Enhance appearance

981. Regulation of most food additives is the responsibility of the:

A. Centers for disease control and prevention

B. United States Department of Agriculture

C. Food and Drug Administration

D. Environmental Protection Agency

982. Antioxidants that prevent rancidity include:

A. Smoke   B. Salt

C. Sugar   D. BHT and BHA

983. Vitamin C and vitamin E, BHA and BHT, and sulfites are all:

A. Antioxidants

B. Flavor enhancers

C. Antimicrobial agents

D. Incidental food additives

984. Nitrite prevents the growth of:

A. C. botulinum   B. C. perfringens

C. S. aureus   D. Yeasts

985. Substances used to preserve foods by lowering the pH are:

A. Smoke and irradiation

B. Vinegar and citric acid

C. Baking powder and soda

D. Salt and sugar

986. The factor that is least important to control in order to limit food-borne illness is:

A. Presence of pesticides

B. Presence of microbes

C. Temperature of food

D. Time of incubation

987. What are the most intensively investigated additives?

A. Flavor enhancers

B. Antimicrobial agents

C. Artificial colors

D. Antioxidants

988. Which of the following body organs does not secrete digestive enzymes?

A. Liver   B. Stomach

C. Pancreas   D. Salivary glands

989. The word organic on a food label is no guarantee that the food is:

A. Pesticide-free

B. Fertilized with manure or vegetable compost

C. Grown without hormones or antibiotics

D. Produced without genetic modification

990. The increasing independence that comes with adolescence can cause nutritional problems, because many adolescents:

A. Have decreased appetites after their major growth spurt has taken place

B. Take medications that diminish the nutritional value of food

C. Spend their food money on illegal drugs

D. Are uninterested in or unaware of the importance of good nutrition

991. What is the main reason for packaging bread in plastic?

A. To maintain air flow

B. To prevent drying out

C. To improve consumer safety

D. To provide marketing opportunities

992. What is meant by product specification in relation to development of food product?

A. A list of consumer expectations

B. A plan of the manufacturing process

C. A measure of the feasibility of the product

D. A description of requirements of production

993. Which of the following is a major advantage of using hazard analysis and critical control point?

A. Low cost of implementation

B. Increased profits and reduced waste

C. Not all staff training

D. More nutritious foods for consumers

994. How do company production facilities impact on product development activities?

A. They determine the production level of the company

B. They reflect the current ecological environment

C. They enable all consumer demands to be met

D. They allow manufacture of completely newer product

995. Carbohydrates, lipids, and proteins all contain carbon, hydrogen, and oxygen. Which one also contains nitrogen?

A. Carbohydrates

B. Proteins

C. Lipids

D. None of the above

996. Pasteurization in milk destroys:

A. Vitamins

B. Bacteria

C. Fat content

D. None of the above

997. Good sources of omega-6 fatty acids are:

A. Sesame, pumpkin, sunflower

B. Potato, guava, pumpkin

C. Sesame, pumpkin, tomato

D. All of the above

998. During ripening fruits produce:

A. Ammonia

B. Oxygen

C. Nitrogen

D. Ethylene gas

999. A fermentation process in which a large amount of salt is used is called:

A. Pickling   B. Boiling

C. Preserving   D. Salting

1000. Sugar processed whole fruit is called:

A. Jelly   B. Pickle

C. Preserve   D. Juice

1001. In 1857, it was proved that all fermentations are the results of microbial activity by:

A. Pasteur   B. Lamark

C. Darwin   D. Mendel

1002. The most common type of fermented cereal is:

A. Yogurt   B. Wheat

C. Rice   D. Bread

1003. The incomplete oxidation and reduction of glucose is:

A. Metabolism

B. Respiration

C. Fermentation

D. Digestion

1004. During alcoholic fermentation, the acetaldehyde is reduced to:

A. Methanol

A. Ethanol

B. Lactose

C. Ascorbic acid

1005. Which of the following is a requisite for a microorganism to be used in fermentation and pickling?

A. Microorganisms must be able to grow on the substrate

B. Organism must have the ability to maintain physiological constancy under growing conditions

C. Desired chemical changes should take place in the required conditions

D. All of the mentioned

1006. Statement 1: What is the use of salt in cheese?

Statement 2: Eyes of the cheese are formed by the growth of certain bacteria. This makes the cheese round.

A. Removing water from cheese surface, false

B. Produces heavy protective rind, false

C. None of the mentioned

D. Neither of the mentioned, false

1007. Pasteurization is applied in which of the following ways?

A. Flash pasteurization and returning to storage tank

B. Flash pasteurization and into the final bottle

C. Pasteurization by heating the filled and sealed bottle

D. All of the mentioned

1008. Which of the following is included in vinegar fermentation?

A. Transform sugar into alcohol, by yeast

B. Change alcohol into acetic acid using vinegar bacteria

C. Transform sugar into alcohol, by yeast and changing alcohol into acetic acid using vinegar bacteria

D. None of the above

1009. The best means of preventing growth of undesirable organisms in fermented juice is to _____

A. Add strong, unpasteurized vinegar after alcoholic fermentation is complete

B. Add sugar

C. All of the mentioned

D. Neither of the above

1010. The rate of conversion of alcohol to acetic acid depends on _____

A. The activity of the organism

B. The amount of alcohol present and the amount of surface exposed per unit of volume

C. The temperature

D. All of the above

1011. Which information is incorrect when it comes to dehydration affecting vitamins?

A. Beta-carotene and B-vitamin do not get affected

B. Vitamin C does not get affected

C. Vitamin C is retained during pickling of vegetables

D. None of the above

1012. Which of the following is false?

A. Many vitamin Bs like vitamin B6 are affected by heating

B. Vitamin C is lost in almost all food processing steps

C. Vitamin C degradation decreases by enzymes and also metals like Cu and Fe

D. Vitamin A is stable in absence of oxygen

1013. Which of the following statements is true with respect to food processing?

A. Sodium is lost during cooking and selenium is volatile and is lost by cooking or processing

B. Vitamins can be removed from food via leaching

C. Mineral losses in food processing are more compared to vitamins

D. Boiling has less mineral losses as compared to steaming

1014. Which of the following operation reduces the dietary fibre content in cereals?

A. Drying

B. Retrogradation

C. Grinding

D. Milling

1015. Which of the following is a food safety tool?

A. Good hygiene practice

B. Hazard analysis critical control point

C. Total quality management

D. All of the above

1016. Hazards affecting food are _____

A. Chemical, biological, physical

B. Additives, colour

C. Pollutants

D. All of the above

1017. Which of the following terms refers to the amount of protein absorbed by the body from a food source?

A. Biological value

B. Limiting value

C. Reference pattern

D. None of the above

1018. Which of the following is incorrect?

A. Controlled cheese ripening is controlling some protein breakdown

B. Proteins form films

C. Egg white cannot be whipped

D. If proteins are over-whipped, the film breaks, foam collapses

1019. Microbial process is advantageous than chemical process.

A. True

B. False

1020. Which of the following is not a product of fermentation?

A. Oxygen

B. Carbon dioxide

C. Ethanol

D. Lactate

1021. Alcoholic fermentation is carried by yeast known as _____

A. *Lactobacillus*

B. *Bacillus*

C. *Saccharomyces cerevisiae*

D. *Escherichia coli*

1022. Which of the following is not a probiotic?

A. Fungi

B. *Saccharomyces cerevisiae*

C. *Escherichia coli*

D. *Lactobacillus*

1023. Vitamin which is not found in fruits and vegetables:

A. Vitamin A   B. Vitamin B_1

C. Vitamin B_6 D. Vitamin B_{12}

1024. Albinism is an important physiological disorder of:

A. Plum   B. Peach

C. Strawberry   D. Cherry

1025. Formation of abscission layer is maturity index of:

A. Tomato   B. Leafy vegetables

C. Onion   D. Melons

1026. In onion pink colour is due to:

A. Anthocyanin   B. Carotene

C. Xanthophyll   D. Quercitin

1027. Vitamin D is chemically known as:

A. Retinol   B. Cobalamin

C. Calciferol   D. Tocopherol

1028. Which of the following is associated with 'browning' disorder?

A. Apple   B. Cabbage

C. Cauliflower   D. Citrus

1029. Louis Pasteur established the modern era of food microbiology in 1857 when he showed that microorganisms cause _____ spoilage:

A. Beer   B. Wine

C. Juice   D. Milk

1030. Which type of fermentation is used to produce yogurt?

A. Mesophilic

B. Thermophilic

C. Therapeutic

D. Yeast-lactic fermentations

1031. Which of the following acid will have higher bacteriostatic effect at a given pH?

A. Acetic acid   B. Tartaric acid

C. Citric acid   D. Maleic acid

1032. Water activity can act as:

A. An intrinsic factor determining the likelihood of microbial proliferation

B. A processing factor

C. An extrinsic factor

D. All of the above

1033. Which one of the following groups of chemicals is not a food nutrient:

A. Proteins   **B. Enzymes**

C. Carbohydrates   D. Vitamins

1034. The chemical reaction that takes place during digestion that involves breakdown with water is:

A. Hydrolysis   B. Hydration

C. Oxidation   D. Regulation

1035. The teeth at the front of the mouth which are used for chopping are called:

A. Incisors   B. Canines

C. Premolars   D. Molars

1036. When proteins are completely broken down the end products are:

A. Glucose molecules

B. Glycerol molecules

C. Amino acids

D. Vitamins

1037. Which one of the following foods does not contain carbohydrate:

A. Potato   B. Sugar

C. Meat   D. Rice

1038. Which one of the following is not a monosaccharide sugar:

A. Glucose   B. Sucrose

C. Fructose   D. Galactose

1039. Which one of the following provides the greatest energy value per gram of nutrient:

A. Carbohydrate   B. Fat

C. Protein   D. Water

1040. When starch is cooked in moist conditions it may:

A. Caramelize   B. Coagulate

C. Gelatinize   D. Oxidize

1041. Which one of the following does not contain fat:

A. Meat   B. Cheese

C. Butter   D. Sugar

1042. The point at which a blue haze is given off from the surface of fat or oil during heating is:

A. The smoke point

B. The melting point

C. The flash point

D. The plastic point

1043. Proteins are made up of:

A. Amino acids

B. Monosaccharides and disaccharides

C. Glycerol units

D. Vitamins and minerals

1044. Which of the following is not a function of amino acids (from protein digestion) in the body?

A. Energy production

B. Regulation of body processes

C. Growth of body tissues

D. Maintenance and repair of body tissues

1045. Which one of the following cooking processes does not rely on coagulation taking place:

A. Frying chips

B. Making yoghurt

C. Whipping cream

D. Boiling an egg.

1046. The best conductor of heat amongst the following is:

A. Iron   B. Stainless steel

C. Aluminium   D. Copper

1047. A method of cooking in which most of the heat transfer is by conduction is:

A. Deep fat frying   B. Shallow frying

C. Grilling   D. Roasting

1048. The transfer of heat in a boiling liquid or hot air in an oven is by:

A. Conduction

B. Convection

C. Infra-red radiation

D. Microwave radiation

1049. Which one of the following materials reflects microwave radiation and therefore should not be used in a microwave oven?

A. Glass

B. China

C. Earthenware

D. Aluminium foil

1050. Which vitamin is most likely to be lost from stewing beef if it is boiled for a long time?

A. Vitamin A   B. Nicotinic acid

C. Vitamin C   D. Vitamin D

1051. In which one of the following methods of cooking is the highest cooking temperature reached?

A. Deep fat frying

B. Boiling

C. Roasting

D. Steaming

1052. Which one of the following methods of cooking is only really suitable for thin tender foods?:

A. Grilling   B. Roasting

C. Steaming   D. Poaching

1053. The temperature at which fat is used for deep frying is likely to be approximately:

A. 150°C   B. 185°C

C. 210°C   D. 225°C

1054. Which one of the following vitamins is *least* affected by cooking and preparation?:

A. Vitamin A   B. The B group

C. Vitamin C   D. Vitamin D

1055. Which one of the following methods of cooking may cause an increase in the nutritional value of the food being cooked?

A. Boiling   B. Steaming

C. Deep frying   D. Roasting

1056. Which one of the following factors does not affect *oxidative* rancidity?

A. Enzymes

B. Oxygen

C. Temperature

D. Ultra-violet light

1057. Most foods should be stored under cool, dry conditions. One of the following groups has a longer life if conditions are *not* too dry:

A. Meat and poultry

B. Fruit and vegetables

C. Cereals

D. Dried fruits

1058. Which one of the following chemicals has been associated with chemical food poisoning?

A. Lead   B. Iron

C. Calcium   D. Phosphorus

1059. The time between consumption of contaminated food and the onset of the symptoms of food poisoning is:

A. Duration of illness

B. The infective period

C. The incubation period

D. The 'carrying' period

1060. Many food processing techniques are based on destroying one of the following bacteria and its spores in particular:

A. *Salmonella*

B. *Clostridium botulinum*

C. *Staphylococcus*

D. *Bacillus cereus*

1061. Only one of the following bacteria produces a toxin (that is, an exotoxin):

A. *Staphylococcus*

B. *Salmonella*

C. *Campylobacter*

D. *Vibrio parahaemolyticus*

1062. Which one of the following organisms causes food poisoning that is often fatal?:

A. *Bacillus cereus*

B. *Staphylococcus*

C. *Clostridium perfringens*

D. *Clostridium botulinum*

1063. Which one of the following bacteria is associated with fish and shellfish?

A. *Bacillus cereus*

B. *Campylobacter*

C. *Salmonella*

D. *Vibrio parahaemolyticus*

1064. Which one of the following foods is not a 'high risk' food?

A. Sausage   B. Trifle

C. Quiche Lorraine D. Pickled onions

1065. *Shigella* causes which one of the following food-borne diseases?

A. Cholera   B. Brucellosis

C. Dysentery   D. Enteric fever

1066. Food is a ____ commodity.

A. Global   B. Local

C. National   D. State

1067. What is the symbol for salt?

A. NaCl   B. H_2O

C. $C_6H_{12}C_6$ D. CO_2

1068. Which of the following is the source of carbohydrates?

A. Animal   B. Plant

C. Human   D. Insect

1069. Which of the complex carbohydrate cannot be digested.

A. Fiber   B. Sugar

C. Cellulose   D. Fat

1070. Which micro-mineral is essential for the production of the thyroid hormones?

A. Calcium   B. Fluorine

C. Iodine   D. Magnesium

1071. Carbohydrates are composed of _____ and _____.

A. Carbon, water

B. Zinc, aluminum

C. Hydrogen, oxygen

D. Gold, calcium

1072. _____percent of the adult body is made up of water.

A. Fifty-five   B. Seventy-five

C. Sixty-five   D. Eighty-five

1073. Most vitamins are measured in _____.

A. Liters   B. Milligrams

C. Grams   D. Kilograms

1074. Naturally occurring _____ play a role in food coloring.

A. Enzymes   B. Pigments

C. Sugars   D. Phenols

1075. _____ or spectrophotometers can be used for measuring transparent foods.
    A. Thermometers
    B. Liquid
    C. Meters
    D. Colorimeters

1076. Fruits and vegetables are graded based on their _____ and _____.
    A. Size, shape
    B. Smell, shape
    C. Color, size
    D. Smell, color

1077. The most common drying method is ____ drying.
    A. Freeze
    B. Spray
    C. Sun or tray drying
    D. Oven

1078. Which one among the following elements/ions is essential in small quantities for development of healthy teeth but causes mottling of the teeth if consumed in higher quantities?
    A. Iron   B. Chloride
    C. Fluoride   D. Potassium

1079. Which one among the following minerals is essential for the transmission of nerve impulses in the nerve fibres of human body?
    A. Calcium   B. Cobalt
    C. Iodine   D. Sodium

1080. Which vitamin is used most commonly to control browning in fruits by enzymes?
    A. K   B. B
    C. C   D. D

1081. Piperine is a compound found in:
    A. Pepper
    B. Turmeric
    C. Cardamom
    D. Cloves

1082. Consider the following statements:
    1. Brinjal is a good source of iron.
    2. Pumpkin is a good source of vitamin A.
    Which of the statements given above is/are correct ?
    A. 1 only   B. 2 only
    C. Both 1 and 2   D. Neither 1 nor 2

1083. Spoilage in food because of microbial activity can be prevented or delayed by:
    A. Prohibiting the entry of microorganisms in food
    B. Physical removal of microorganisms
    C. Hindering the activity of microorganisms
    D. All of the above

1084. The growth of aerobic food spoilage and pathogenic microorganisms can be suppressed by:
    A. Humectants
    B. Exhausting
    C. Both A and B
    D. None of the above

1085. The target microorganism in canning is:
    A. *Clostridium botulinum*
    B. *Streptococcus thermophillus*
    C. PA 3679
    D. *Lactobacillus bulgaricus*

1086. Pasteurization is the heat treatment designed primarily to kill:
    A. Vegetable forms of microorganisms
    B. All form of microorganisms
    C. Spore
    D. None of the above

1087. In bread manufacturing, alcoholic fermentation is carried out by:
    A. *Streptococcus thermophillus*
    B. *Saccharomyces cerevisiae*
    C. *S. carlsbergensis*
    D. *Lactobacillus bulgaricus*

1088. *Clostridium botulinum* mainly result in spoilage of _____ foods.
A. High acid food
B. Acidic food
C. Medium acid food
D. Low acid food

1089. Any change that renders food unfit for human consumption is called:
A. Processing
B. Spoilage
C. Deterioration
D. Preservation

1090. Food intoxication is the ingestion of:
A. Toxin produced by microorganism
B. Toxin producing microorganism
C. None of the above
D. Both of these

1091. Carbohydrates are also known as _____
A. Hydrates of carbon
B. Carbonates
C. Glycolipids
D. Polysaccharides

1092. Class of carbohydrate which cannot be hydrolyzed further, is known as?
A. Disaccharides   B. Polysaccharides
C. Proteoglycan   D. Monosaccharide

1093. Which class of carbohydrates is considered as non-sugar?
A. Monosaccharides
B. Disaccharides
C. Polysaccharides
D. Oligosaccharides

1094. Mark the INCORRECT statement about sugar alcohol?
A. Addition of -itol as a suffix
B. A linear molecule that cannot cyclize
C. Carbonyl groups reduced to a hydroxyl group
D. Terminal –OH group oxidizes

1095. Name the major storage form of carbohydrates in animals?
A. Cellulose   B. Chitin
C. Glycogen   D. Starch

1096. Biomolecules simply refer to as "Staff of life" in the given _____
A. Protein
B. Lipids
C. Carbohydrate
D. Vitamins

1097. The simplest carbohydrate is _____
A. Dihydroxy acetone
B. Glyceraldehyde
C. Glucose
D. Gulose

1098. The first food designated as a Food for Specified Health Use (FOSHU) in Japan was:
A. An oat bran-enriched breakfast cereal
B. A plant sterol-enriched margarine
C. An isotonic sports drink
D. A hypoallergenic rice grain

1099. Vitamin D may reduce the risk of all but one of these. Which one?
A. Bone loss
B. Colon cancer
C. Gum disease
D. Irritable bowel syndrome

1100. Which is least likely to reduce your risk of diabetes?
A. Whole-grain cereal
B. Nuts
C. Alcoholic beverages
D. Orange juice

1101. Which is least likely to lower your risk of colon cancer?
A. Lean meat
B. Whole-grain bread
C. Low-fat milk
D. A multivitamin

1102. Which is least likely to lower your risk of brittle bones (osteoporosis)?
    A. Low-fat yogurt   B. Collard greens
    C. Olive oil   D. Multivitamin

1103. Meat eaters have a higher risk of all but one of these diseases. Which one?
    A. Osteoarthritis   B. Diabetes
    C. Gout   D. Colon cancer

1104. Canning of fruits and vegetables is a _____ process
    A. Cold   B. Heat
    C. Irradiation   D. Microwave

1105. Green tea is _____
    A. Orthodox tea
    B. Fermented tea
    C. Unfermented tea
    D. Semi-fermented tea

1106. Low temperature storage of potatoes results in:
    A. Sweet
    B. Have more sugar
    C. Have more starch
    D. Both A and B

1107. Scalding of vegetables is a:
    A. Freezing treatment
    B. Irradiation
    C. Fermentation
    D. Heat treatment

1108. Corn syrup is a mixture of:
    A. Dextrose and maltose
    B. Dextrose and galactose
    C. Galactose and maltose
    D. Glucose and galactose

1109. Strong flour is recommended for:
    A. Cookies
    B. Cakes
    C. Bread
    D. All of the above

1110. Which of the following is not the property of the fermented food?
    A. Highly nutritious
    B. Toxic
    C. Antitoxicity
    D. Antinutrient

1111. Which of the following is produced by fermenting soybeans?
    A. Yogurt
    B. Kombucha
    C. Miso
    D. Jiangs

1112. Probiotics are used in the prevention of _____
    A. Cardiac disease
    B. Hypertension
    C. Digestive tract disease
    D. Lungs infection

1113. Sauerkraut is _____
    A. A cauliflower
    B. A potato
    C. A cabbage
    D. A tomato

1114. You should eat fruits and vegetables because:
    A. They contain fiber, which helps keep your digestive system healthy
    B. They give you energy
    C. They contain vitamins and minerals that help you stay healthy
    D. All of the above

1115. Vitamin A is important for good eyesight, helps your body fight infection, and keeps your skin and hair healthy. Which of the following foods have the most vitamin A?
    A. Meats
    B. Breads
    C. Deep yellow or orange fruits and vegetables
    D. Candy

1116. If you eat too much fat, you are more likely to gain weight and develop heart disease. Which of these foods contain the least amount of fat?

A. Breads   B. Fruits

C. Vegetables   D. Both B and C

1117. When the food is directly given in the veins, it is called _____ nutrition.

A. Parenteral   B. Enteral

C. Intravenous   D. Saline

1118. Vitamin C helps your body fight disease by maintaining a strong immune system. Which food has more vitamin C?

A. Milk   B. Oranges

C. Broccoli   D. Bread

1119. Digestion of your food begins in your mouth when you chew your food and expose it to saliva. It then travels through the rest of your digestive tract. Fiber is needed to keep your digestive tract healthy. Which of these foods will provide the most fiber per serving?

A. Fresh fruits and vegetables

B. Cheese

C. Chicken

D. Orange juice

1120. Calcium is needed to keep bones strong. Which vegetable contains a significant amount of calcium?

A. Squash   B. Sweet potato

C. Broccoli   D. Green onion

1121. Vitamin A is made of the elements lutien and indoles. In which food would you find the most vitamin A?

A. Spinach   B. Grapes

C. Bananas   D. Lettuce

1122. Fiber is needed to keep your digestive system working properly. It is especially important to the health of your intestines. Which of these foods has the most fiber?

A. Milk   B. White bread

C. Raisins   D. White rice

1123. The energy your body needs to allow your muscles to work comes from the food you eat.

A. True

B. False

1124. Eating non-nutritious food will make you _____.

A. Tired

B. Overweight

C. Not perform well

D. All of the above

1125. To maintain good health, you should eat healthy foods, drink plenty of water, exercise regularly, and _____.

A. Sleep less

B. Get plenty of rest

C. Sleep only when you're really tired

D. Drink plenty of sports drinks

1126. Which of the following factor of food is considered as intrinsic factor from food safety point of view:

A. Water activity (a_w)

B. Relative humidity

C. Temperature

D. Vapour pressure

1127. The person suffering from which of the following disease can work inside food processing industry:

A. Diarrhoea

B. Vomiting

C. Excessive hair fall

D. None of the above

1128. Which of the following factors contributing to food poisoning:

A. Food prepared too far in advance

B. Cooling food too slowly

C. Not re-heating food to high enough temperatures

D. All of the above

1129. Who among the following is most at risk to food poisoning:

A. Elder people

B. Toddlers, babies, and pregnant women

C. Individuals who are already unwell

D. All of the above

1130. The term 'due diligence' means:

A. Food is contaminated and not safe to eat

B. Food is contaminated but safe to eat in due course of time

C. A food is prepared doing everything to safeguard consumer health

D. A food is prepared got contaminated and re-processed to remove contamination

1131. Which of the following is correct procedure for storage of food products:

A. Raw material and cooked food can be kept at same place

B. It is better to keep food product with outer package in the storage

C. Follow the principle first in first out (FIFO)

D. Cleaning material such as detergents should not be stored in a separate area

1132. What can be potential hazards in refrigerated storage:

A. Bacterial growth

B. Cross contamination

C. Food beyond date marking

D. All of the above

1133. Which of the following is not ideal regarding the refrigerated storage:

A. Maintain temperatures of 0–5°C

B. Do not place hot foods directly in the refrigerator as this will cause the temperature of the refrigerator to rise above 5°C

C. Do not defrost and clean the fridge or freezer box regularly

D. Do not overload the fridge as cold air needs to be allowed to circulate

1134. Which of the following is not recommended practice related to "Use by dates" in pre-packed food:

A. It is found on high risk foods likely to cause food poisoning

B. It is a good practice to sell food past its "use by date"

C. The food should be disposed of immediately once it is past its "use by date"

D. None of the following

1135. Which of the following is not recommended practice related to "Best before dates"—indicates the date until the food may be in its best condition.

A. These usually appear on canned, dried and frozen products

B. It is NOT an automatic offence to sell products past their "best before dates", but their quality might be compromised

C. Both of the above

D. None of the above

1136. What are the pillars of Good Agricultural Practices (GAP)

A. Economic viability; environmental sustainability; social acceptability; food safety and quality

B. Economic viability; social acceptability; food safety and quality

C. Social acceptability; food safety and quality

D. Economic viability; environmental sustainability

1137. Food laws are classified in:

A. Mandatory standards and voluntary standards

B. Preventive standards and hygienic standards

C. Safety standards and security standards

D. General standards and potential standards

1138. Which of the following are voluntary standards

A. Food Safety and Standards Act, 2006
B. The Essential Commodities Act, 1955
C. The Insecticides Act, 1968
D. Codex Alimentarius Standards

1139. Which of the following are mandatory standards

A. Codex Alimentarius Standards
B. BIS standards and specifications
C. Consumer Protection Act, 1986
D. Food Safety and Standards Act, 2006

1140. The aim behind FSSAI establishment was/ were:

A. To establish a single reference point for all matters relating to food safety and standards
B. To move from multi-level, multi-departmental control to a single line of command
C. To establish an independent statutory authority
D. All of the above

1141. What is/are the mandate behind the establishment of FSSAI, 2006:

A. To lay down science based standards for food articles
B. To regulate their manufacture, storage, distribution, sale and import
C. To ensure availability of safe and whole-some food for human consumption
D. All of the above

1142. How much women candidates are necessary in "Composition of Food Authority" in FSSAI

A. Out of twenty-two members, three shall be women
B. Out of twenty-two members, two shall be women
C. Out of twenty-two members, one-third shall be women

D. Out of twenty-two members, one-fourth shall be women

1143. How many referral food laboratories are there in FSSAI

A. 4   B. 5
C. 36   D. 39

1144. How much time it will take to get FSSAI license once all the documentation and fees paying is done

A. Within 30 days   B. Within 60 days
C. Within 80 days   D. Within 10 days

1145. In which format licence is issued?

A. Format A   B. Format B
C. Format C   D. Format D

1146. Which portion of wheat is rich in starch?

A. Endosperm   B. Bran
C. Germ   D. None

1147. Which portion of wheat is rich in sugar?

A. Endosperm   B. Bran
C. Germ   D. Aleurone layer

1148. If extraction is done at the _____ of the solvent, it is called _____

A. Melting point, decoction
B. Boiling point, decoction
C. Melting point, leaching
D. Boiling point, leaching

1149. Oil seed cakes are obtained by _____

A. Solvent extraction
B. Mechanical pressing
C. None of the mentioned
D. Solvent extraction and mechanical pressing

1150. Which among the following factors does not affect extraction?

A. Solubility of solute in the solvent
B. Degree of agitation
C. Concentration difference
D. None of the mentioned

1151. Who developed the process of canning?
   A. Nicolas Appert
   B. Louis Pasteur
   C. Norman Borlaug
   D. Water Hesse

1152. Mold inhibitor used in bread is:
   A. Calcium carbonate
   B. Sodium chloride
   C. Sodium/calcium propionate
   D. None of these

1153. Bitterness in colocasia is due to:
   A. Calcium carbonate
   B. Calcium chloride
   C. Potassium oxalate
   D. Calcium oxalate

1154. Food processing in India is concentrated in which sector, maximum?
   A. Organized sector
   B. Unorganized sector
   C. Small scale
   D. None of the mentioned

1155. Which among these is a factor for processed food in India?
   A. Changing lifestyles
   B. Food habits
   C. Organized food retail
   D. All of the above

1156. Statement 1: There will be a shift of demand snacks, convenience food and organic and diet food.
   Statement 2: High taxation is a constraint for the food processing industry.
   A. True, false   B. True, true
   C. False, false   D. False, true

1157. Which of the following is NOT a function of a food additive _____
   A. To maintain product consistency
   B. Maintain nutritive value
   C. Controlling acidity/alkalinity
   D. None of the mentioned

1158. Statement 1: Food additives are divided into direct and indirect types.
   Statement 2: Direct food additives become a part of the food during packaging. These are in trace amounts.
   A. True, false   B. True, true
   C. False, false   D. False, true

1159. The 'WFP' stands for:
   A. Wild Food Program
   B. World Food Program
   C. Wild fire protection
   D. Wild fauna protection

1160. The ulcer of the stomach is also known as:
   A. Corneal ulcer
   B. Venous ulcer
   C. Gastric ulcer
   D. Peptic ulcer

1161. Which of the following is true about bacteria?
   A. Bacteria multiplies and grows faster in warm environments.
   B. Bacteria needs air to survive.
   C. Every type of bacteria can give people food poisoning.
   D. By freezing food you can kill bacteria.

1162. Food contaminated with food poisoning bacteria would:
   A. Look different
   B. Smell badly
   C. Look and taste normal
   D. Generally speaking food poisoning bacteria cannot be smelled, tasted or seen (except with the aid of a microscope) on food

1163. In a place of work, the best way to dry your hands after washing them is to:
   A. Use a cotton towel
   B. Just shake excess water away
   C. Use a air dryer
   D. Use a paper towel

1164. Agencies involved behind "Plant Quarantine (regulation of import into India) Order, 2003"

A. Ministry of Health and Family Welfare

B. Ministry of Food Processing Industries

C. Department of Agriculture and Cooperation

D. Directorate General of Health Services

1165. _____ is an important mineral nutrient

A. Hydrogen   B. Nitrogen

C. Oxygen   D. Carbon

1166. _____ is not a trace element

A. Sodium   B. Boron

C. Carbon   D. Zinc

1167. _____ is a trace element

A. Phosphorus   B. Carbon

C. Magnesium   D. Sodium

1168. All the following techniques are household preservation technique *except:*

A. Smoking   B. Lyophilisation

C. Dehydration   D. Salting

1169. About half of your diet should be made up of _____.

A. Grains and vegetables

B. Fruits and milk

C. Milk and cheese

D. Fats and sugars

1170. According to the my Pyramind food guidance system, a person should obtain most of their fat from _____.

A. Beef, chicken, and fish

B. Vegetables oils, nuts, and fish

C. Fats, oils, and sweets

D. Milk, yogurt, and cheese

1171. This food group is our body's best source of energy?

A. Meat group

B. Fats, oils and sweets

C. Breads and cereals

D. Milk and cheese

1172. Which of these is added to the food label because people sometimes do not eat enough of this?

A. Fat   B. Calcium

C. Sodium   D. Cholesterol

1173. The bread, cereal, rice and pasta group is a good source of _____.

A. Carbohydrate

B. Vitamin C

C. Calcium

D. Vitamin D

1174. Foods from the meat, poultry, fish dry beans, eggs and nuts group are an important source of _____?

A. Iron   B. Fiber

C. Beta carotene   D. Calcium

1175. The milk, cheese and yogurt group are important for _____.

A. Strong bones

B. Teeth

C. Muscles

D. All of the above

1176. Which of the following is a reducing sugar?

A. Starch   B. Lactose

C. Fructose   D. Sucrose

1177. Malic acid is the predominant acid present in:

A. Plum   B. Peach

C. Citrus   D. Mango

1178. Pyruvic acid is the end product of:

A. Electron transport system

B. Phosphate metabolism

C. Glycolysis

D. Fat metabolism

1179. Exhausting of cans is done to:

A. Sterilize the cans

B. Raise the sugar contents

C. Remove the acid

D. Expel the entrapped air in the contents

1180. Pasteurization is done to kill:

     A. Selective microorganism

     B. All the microorganism

     C. Yeast

     D. Yeast and its spores

1181. BOD stands for:

     A. Biological oxygen demand

     B. Biochemical oxygen demand

     C. Biodegradable oxygen demand

     D. Biowaste of diesel

1182. Calcium is used in human body for:

     A. Synthesis of bones

     B. Recovery of bicarbonate

     C. Utilisation of sulphate

     D. Synthesis of amino acids

1183. Lacquering of tin cans is done to:

     A. Prevent discolouration of products

     B. To make the can attractive

     C. Kill the microorganism

     D. Expell the air

1184. Out of these which is/are irradiated for sterilization purpose:

     A. Spices   B. Potatoes

     C. Rice   D. All of these

1185. Cold sterilization is also called:

     A. Freezing   B. Chilling

     C. Vacuum cooling D. Irradiation

1186. Food is a hot commodity! If we produce food that does not get eaten, what else is wasted?

     A. Wildlife habitat

     B. Water

     C. Energy

     D. All of the above

1187. What food, when wasted, represents the biggest waste of energy?

     A. Milk   B. Poultry

     C. Corn   D. Beef

1188. Maximum carbohydrates are obtained from:

     A. Whole grain food

     B. Fatty fish

     C. Plant oil

     D. Nuts

1189. The sources of proteins includes:

     A. Fish   B. Poultry

     C. Eggs   D. All of them

1190. Fiber helps to reduce the risk of all of the following *except* _____.

     A. Cancer

     B. Heart disease

     C. Diabetes

     D. Diverticulitis

1191. Which of the following is called metabolic regulators?

     A. Vitamins and minerals

     B. Vitamins and water

     C. Minerals and roughage

     D. Carbohydrates and vitamins

1192. What is the formula for glucose?

     A. $C_6H_{12}O_6$ B. $C_6H_6O_{12}$

     C. $C_6H_6O_6$ D. $C_{12}H_6O_{11}$

1193. Which of the following carbohydrates give the instant source of energy?

     A. Glucose

     B. Fructose

     C. Cellulose

     D. Starch

1194. The human body uses carbohydrates in the form of_____.

     A. Glucose   B. Glycogen

     C. Starch   D. Enzymes

1195. In which form body stores glucose?

     A. Cellulose

     B. Starch

     C. Glycogen and cellulose

     D. Glycogen

1196. **Which organ of human body stores glucose in the form of glycogen?**

    A. Lungs

    B. Liver and muscles

    C. Stomach and muscles

    D. Small intestine

1197. **The safety of which of the following substances must be demonstrated prior to their introduction into food?**

    A. Pesticide chemicals

    B. Substances migrating from food packaging

    C. Colour additives

    D. All of the above

1198. **The model for food safety standards is based on a system called:**

    A. HACCP—hazard analysis and critical control points

    B. GMP—good manufacturing practices

    C. PHP—public health plan

    D. Scientific studies and government regulation

1199. **Food Safety is of particular importance for which of the following groups?**

    A. Children under the age of six

    B. Adults over the age of sixty five

    C. People with immune deficiencies

    D. All of the above

1200. **For any workstation within a kitchen, the following article(s) should always be found:**

    A. Plastic hand gloves

    B. Red bucket filled with diluted bleach water

    C. Head gear

    D. All of the above

1201. **To avoid foods spoiling in the refrigerator or freezer, which of the following actions is always recommended?**

    A. Placing the oldest product on top of newer product

    B. Ordering foods for a few days at a time only

    C. Placing a date of arrival on all foods

    D. Smelling the food to make sure it is fresh

1202. **Food prepared at home or in an unlicensed kitchen are:**

    A. Illegal

    B. Cheaper

    C. Tasty

    D. To be served immediately

1203. **What is a substitute for proper hand washing?**

    A. Sanitizers   B. Gloves

    C. Tongs   D. None of these

1204. **Which of the following are potentially hazardous foods?**

    A. Potato, chips, bread and crackers

    B. Hamburgers, cooked beans, cut melons

    C. Candy bars

    D. Cereal and dry pasta

1205. **How common are food spoilage micro-organisms?**

    A. They are extremely rare

    B. Almost none of our foods contain them

    C. Our foods contain them

    D. Almost all of our foods contain them

1206. **The most common organisms causing food spoilage are bacteria:**

    A. Yeast and insects

    B. Yeasts and molds

    C. Molds and insects

    D. Insects and parasites

1207. **By keeping food cold the growth of microorganisms is:**

    A. Increased

    B. Not changed

    C. Minimized

    D. Stopped and they are killed

1208. Workers should not handle food or eating and drinking utensils when they have or recently had any of the following symptoms:

A. Vomiting, diarrhea, fever, sore throat with fever, jaundice, infected cuts

B. Runny nose, sneezing, cough, congestion, cold symptoms

C. Both A and B

D. None of the above

1209. Food workers should wash their hands after which of the following:

A. Coughing, sneezing, scratching, wiping nose, cleaning

B. Touching exposed body parts, handling raw animal food, handling money

C. Before putting on disposable gloves or after using the rest room

D. All of the above

1210. Disposable gloves should be worn by workers handling which foods:

A. Raw chicken being placed in a deep fryer

B. Sandwich bread for immediate service to customers

C. Both A and B

D. None of the above

1211. For simplicity and safety, all raw poultry, beef, fish and meat should be cooked to what minimum temperature:

A. 165°F (74°C)

B. 185°F (85°C)

C. 212°F (100°C)

D. None of the above

1212. All foods that must be refrigerated should be held at or below what maximum temperature:

A. 51°F (11°C)

B. 41°F (5°C)

C. 32°F (0°C)

D. None of the above

1213. Examples of cross-contamination are:

A. Raw chicken is processed on cutting board then lettuce is sliced on same surface

B. Food worker handles raw meat then assembles sandwich without washing hands

C. Liquids from raw hamburger drip onto vegetables for salad

D. All of the above

1214. Examples of how to rapidly cool food include:

A. Portioning large quantities of foods into smaller units by slicing and pouring

B. Using metal rather than plastic containers

C. Ensuring vigorous air circulation around food

D. All of the above

1215. Agmark act 1937 comes under

A. Department of Consumer Affairs, Govt. of India

B. Department of Agriculture and Cooperation

C. Department of Marketing and Inspection

D. Department of Legal Meterology

1216. What is an example of Biological Hazard

A. Salmonella   B. Dirt

C. Cleaners   D. Antibiotics

1217. What is HACCP system for?

A. Physical, chemical and biological Hazards

B. A systematic analysis of all steps and regular monitoring of the control points

C. Identifying the CCPs, including their location, procedure and process

D. Accurately monitoring food hygiene hazards

1218. SPS under WTO stands for:

A. Standards, prevention and specification

B. Sanitary and ohytosanitary measures

C. Specifications for products and supplements

D. Safety and prevention of sickness

1219. Food Safety and Standards Act, 2006, passed by Indian parliament and notified on:

A. 23rd July 2006

B. 23rd June 2006

C. 23rd August 2006

D. 23rd November 2006

1220. ISO 19011:2011 Quality Management System deals with:

A. Specifications with guidance for use

B. Guidelines for performance improvements

C. Customer satisfaction

D. Guidelines for quality and or environmental management system auditing

1221. Coffee is adulterated with:

A. Saw dust   B. Chicory

C. Ghee   D. All of these

1222. Sugar and salt act as preservatives by:

A. Killing microorganisms directly

B. Increasing the acid content of food

C. Increasing the water content of food

D. Binding water so it is not available for microorganisms

1223. Out of these, which bacterium is found in processed/cured meat?

A. Moraxella   B. Alcaligenes

C. Pseudomonas   D. Lactobacillus

1224. How many acts are repealed by Food Safety and Standards Act, 2006?

A. 4   B. 7

C. 5   D. 8

1225. Currently standards are present for which of the following?

i. Packaged drinking water

ii. Piped drinking water

iii. Well and canal water

A. i, ii   B. i

C. i, iii   D. All of the above

1226. Which of the following is/are true about potassium bromate?

i. Potassium bromate is a category 2B carcinogen

ii. Potassium bromate increases dough strength, leads to higher rising and uniform finish to baked products

iii. Food Safety and Standards Authority of India (FSSAI) permits them up to 50 parts per million

A. i, iii   B. i, ii

C. ii, iii   D. All of the above

1227. The mandate assigned to the food authority is:

A. Laying down science based standards for articles of food

B. To facilitate food safety

C. To regulate manufacture, store, distribution, sale and import of food

D. All of the above

1228. How many scientific panels have been constituted in food authority?

A. 16   B. 7

C. 9   D. 5

1229. Benefits of implementing HACCP/ISO 22000:

A. A preventive approach to food safety

B. Reduce the need for and cost of end product testing

C. Can help identify process improvements and reduce customer complaints

D. All of the above

1230. Which of these is not an International Standards and Statutes

A. Codex Alimentarius Commission (CAC)

B. European Union Standards (EU standards)

C. Food and Agriculture Organization (FAO)

D. Bureau of Indian Standards

1231. FSSAI is located in 5 regions with head office located at:
   A. Hyderabad   B. Mumbai
   C. Bangalore   D. New Delhi

1232. ISO 9001: 2008 quality management systems deals with
   A. Fundamentals and vocabulary
   B. Guidelines for performance improvements
   C. Customer satisfaction
   D. Requirements for quality management

1233. As per the definition for food under the Food Act in India, food does not include
   A. Alcoholic beverages
   B. Caffeinated beverages
   C. Chewing gum
   D. Chewing tobacco

1234. As per Food Safety and Standards Act, FSMS stands for:
   A. Food Security Management System
   B. Food Safety Management System
   C. Food Standards Management System
   D. Food Safety Mechanization System

1235. As per Section 3 of Food Safety and Standards Act, 2006, if food article sold in the market contains any inferior or cheaper substances whether wholly or partly which is injurious to health then such products can be called:
   A. Sub-standard
   B. Unsafe
   C. Misbranded
   D. Partly sub-standard

1236. As per section 22 of FSS Act, 2006, foods for special dietary uses or functional foods or nutraceuticals or health supplements does not include:
   A. Botanical extracts
   B. Vitamin supplements
   C. Parenterals
   D. Probiotics

1237. Food Authority may notify laboratories and research institutions accredited by NABL or any such accreditation agencies, wherein NABL stands for:
   A. National Accreditation Board for Laboratories
   B. National Accreditation Board for Testing Laboratories
   C. National Accreditation Board for Calibration Laboratories
   D. National Accreditation Board for Testing and Calibration Laboratories

1238. Act/order which is not deemed after implementation of Food Safety and Standards Act, 2006:
   A. Fruit Products Order 1955
   B. Prevention of Food Adulteration Act 1954
   C. Milk and Milk Products Order 1992
   D. Standard Weights and Measures Act 1976

1239. Which of the following requires special cleaning procedure in a food testing laboratory?
   A. Broken thermometer
   B. Broken pipette
   C. Ethanol spills
   D. HOCl spills

1240. The normal specific gravity of milk at 27°C ranges from _____ to _____.
   A. 1.028 – 1.038
   B. 1.023 – 1.033
   C. 1.023 – 2.028
   D. 1.028 – 1.033

1241. Iodine concentration used to detect the added starch in milk is _____
   A. 0.5%   B. 1%
   C. 1.5%   D. 2%

1242. LOD of iodine solution method for detection of added starch _____
   A. 0.01%   B. 0.02%
   C. 0.03%   D. 0.05%

1243. Reagent used for the detection of cellulose in milk and milk products:

A. I_2 – ZnCl solution

B. I_2 – TnCl solution

C. I_2 – MnCl solution

D. I_2 – SnCl solution

1244. Cellulose in the milk cannot be detected using iodine–zinc chloride solution in the presence of _____

A. Added cane sugar

B. Added palm sugar

C. Added starch

D. Added glucose

1245. What is Seliwanoff's reagent _____

A. 0.1% resorchinol solution

B. 0.5% resorchinol solution

C. 1.0% resorchinol solution

D. 0.05% resorchinol solution

1246. What is maltodextrin?

A. Enzymatic derivative of cellulose

B. Enzymatic derivative of hemi-cellulose

C. Enzymatic derivative of starch

D. Enzymatic derivative of glycogen

1247. Reagent used to detect the added urea in milk _____

A. Phosphomolybdic acid

B. p-Dimethylaminobenzaldehyde

C. Alpha naphthol

D. Resorchinol

1248. Which of the following is not an adulterant in milk?

A. Water

B. NaCl

C. Urea

D. None of the above

1249. Presence of nitrates in milk indicates adulteration with _____

A. Urea

B. Pond water

C. Oil

D. Detergent

1250. Rosalic acid test is used to detect _____

A. Detergents

B. Oil

C. Urea

D. Sodium carbonate

1251. Formaldehyde is naturally present in which of the following _____

A. Milk

B. Fish

C. Meat

D. Water

1252. What is formalin?

A. 40% formaldehyde

B. 100% formaldehyde

C. 50% formaldehyde

D. 10% formaldehyde

1253. Which of the following is not a permitted preservative in food products?

A. Formalin

B. Benzoic acid

C. Sorbic acid

D. Acetic acid

1254. Which of the following is an adulterant in sesame oil?

A. Palmolein oil

B. Groundnut oil

C. Coconut oil

D. All the above

1255. High acid value in oils is an indicator for _____

A. Degree of unsaturation

B. Degree of saturation

C. Rancidity

D. Polarity

1256. Which of the following is not an edible oil _____

A. Rape seed oil

B. Palmolein

C. Cotton seed oil

D. Castor seed oil

1257. Adulterants used in turmeric powder includes:

A. Lead chromate, chalk powder, metanil yellow, anilline dyes

B. Lead chromate, chalk powder, metanil yellow, anilline dyes, starch

C. Lead chromate, chalk powder, metanil yellow, anilline dyes, starch, brick powder

D. Lead chromate

1258. Which synthetic food colour used as an adulterant in chilli powder?

A. Sudan III   B. Sunset yellow
C. Rhodamine B   D. Orange

1259. Which one of the following is not a monocotyledon?

A. Turmeric   B. Pepper
C. Papaya   D. Grass

1260. Which of the following pathogenic bacteria shall be absent in turmeric powder?

A. *Shigella*
B. *Salmonella*
C. *Staphylococcus aureus*
D. *E. coli*

1261. Ginger is a:

A. Rhizome   B. Tuber
C. Root   D. All of the above

1262. Lactoferrin is an iron binding _____ that is inhibitory to a number of food borne bacteria.

A. Lipoprotein   B. Glycoprotein
C. Lactoprotein   D. Dipeptide

1263. Milk is deficient in one of the following vitamin _____

A. A   B. B complex
C. C   D. D

1264. Yellow colour in cow milk is due to _____

A. Xanthophyll   B. Riboflavin
C. Carotene   D. Bixin

1265. Lactose is composed of D-galactose and D-glucose linked through _____

A. Alpha (5–8)   B. Alpha (1–4)
C. Beta (5–8)   D. Beta (1–4)

1266. The following is not a potent anti-oxidant _____

A. Capsaicin
B. Nordihydroguaieretic acid
C. Tertiary butyl hydroquinone
D. Casoxin

1267. Sorbates and benzoates preservatives are most active at following pH of food system:

A. 7   B. 9
C. 4.5   D. 2

1268. Incorporation of soy flour to wheat flour would enrich the bread with following constituent _____

A. Lysine   B. Fiber
C. Lactose   D. Iron

1269. Amongst derivatives of lactose, _____ is the anomer of lactose.

A. Lactobionic acid B. Lactulose
C. Epilactose   D. Lactitol

1270. Gluten is very unique food present in _____

A. Barley   B. Oat
C. Rice   D. Wheat

1271. In Kjeldahl method of Nitrogen estimation, indicator comprises _____

A. Methyl red + methylene blue
B. Methyl orange + bromophenol blue
C. Methyl orange + methylene blue
D. Methyl red + bromophenol blue

1272. Inhibitory effect of milk peptides on the angiotensin converting enzyme (ACE inhibition) is used for making products for controlling _____

A. Cholesterol   B. Hypertension
C. Osteoporosis   D. Immune functions

1273. Which of the following is not a natural colour?

A. Cyanidine 3 glucoside

B. Chlorophyll

C. Sunset yellow

D. Annatto

1274. The principal acid formed on heating of lactose at temperature above 100°C.

A. Oxalic acid   B. Lactic acid

C. Lactobionic acid D. Formic acid

1275. Linoleic and linolenic acid are not synthesized in the mammary gland and have to be supplied in the diet; they are therefore called _____

A. Unsaturated fatty acids

B. Essential fatty acids

C. Polyenoic acids

D. None of the above

1276. Retrogradation can lead to _____ to expel water from polymer network.

A. Gelling

B. Syneresis

C. Dextrinization

D. Annealing

1277. Increase in volume, viscosity and translucency of starch granules when they are heated in a liquid is called _____

A. Retrogradation

B. Dextrinization

C. Inversion

D. Gelatinization

1278. Trypsin hydrolyses a peptide bond on the carboxyl side of:

A. Leucine   B. Phenylalanine

C. Arginine   D. Proline

1279. Dominant sugar presents in hemicelluloses is _____

A. Ribose   B. Ribulose

C. Xylulose   D. Xylose

1280. Celiac disease is a manifestation of _____

A. Lactose intolerance

B. Tropical sprue

C. Chronic constipation

D. Gluten intolerance

1281. Element that acts as an antioxidant and have synergistic effect with vitamin E is:

A. Selenium   B. Iron

C. Copper   D. Iodine

1282. Naturally occurring form of amino acid in proteins:

A. L-amino acids only

B. D-amino acids only

C. Both L and D amino acids

D. None of these

1283. Conversion of casein to paracasein requires _____

A. Protease and renin

B. Papain and renin

C. Magnesium ions and renin

D. Calcium ions and renin

1284. Identify the correct statement:

A. Quality control is a product focused concept while quality assurance is a process focused concept

B. Quality control is a process focused concept while quality assurance is a product focused concept

C. Quality control and quality assurance are interchangeable in present ISO era

D. None of the above is correct

1285. Why is HACCP, a prerequisite and important to a food manufacture?

A. It prioritizes and controls potential hazards in food production

B. Public health protection is strengthened as it controls major food risks

C. Consumer assure that the products are as safe

D. All of the Above

1286. A Food-borne infection occurs when?

A. The microorganism itself is ingested with the food and the person already has a cold or some other virus

B. The microorganism itself is ingested with the food, establishes itself in the host body, multiplies to significant enough members to cause illness

C. The microorganism itself is ingested with the food, and produces a toxin either in the food or host body. The toxin causes illness.

D. Raw animal products come into contact with the food handlers open sore or lesion

1287. Maillard reaction products which are mutagenic and carcinogenic in nature and are formed during food processing involves?

A. Acid and protein

B. Amino acids and reducing sugar

C. Protein, moisture and heat

D. None of the above

1288. Which of the following process creates free radicals in the food which can destroy the cell membrane and attack DNA and proteins, thus preventing microorganisms growth?

A. Pasteurization

B. Reduction

C. Irradiation

D. Oxidation

1289. Lathyrism is caused by:

A. Argemone seeds

B. Kesari dal

C. Aflatoxin

D. Heavy metals

1290. Urea is added to milk to increase-

A. Thickness

B. Shelf-life

C. Nitrogen content

D. Brightness

1291. Nutraceutical is a food, food component that has been shown to:

A. Curative effect on disease

B. Beneficial effect on health beyond basic nutrition

C. Preventive effect on diseases

D. Antiaging effect

1292. The most common symptom of food-borne illness is:

A. Kidney failure   B. Diarrhea

C. Skin rash   D. Headache

1293. Which of the following groups has the lowest risk for food-borne illness?

A. Young adults

B. Elderly

C. Infants

D. None of the above

1294. Which of the following is correct procedure for storage of food products?

A. Raw material and cooked food can be kept at same place

B. It is better to keep food product with outer package in the storage

C. Follow the principle first in first out (FIFO)

D. Cleaning material such as detergents should not be stored in a separate area

1295. The person suffering from which of the following disease can work inside food processing industry?

A. Diarrhea

B. Vomiting

C. Excessive hair fall

D. None of the above

1296. Food laws are classified into:

A. Mandatory standards and voluntary standards

B. Preventive standards and hygienic standards

C. Safety standards and security standards

D. General standards and potential standards

1297. The two parts of HACCP include:

A. Hazard analysis and critical control points

B. Health analysis and critical control points

C. Hope analysis and critical control points

D. Hazardous analysis and critical control points

1298. The first synthetic sweetening agent used was:

A. Saccharin

B. Cyclamates

C. Aspartame

D. Sucralose

1299. Term used for addition of nutrients to food that were not originally present.

A. Food enrichment

B. Food fortification

C. Food diversification

D. None of these

1300. Which dietary component helps to maintain a constant body temperature in our body?

A. Roughage

B. Water

C. Vitamins

D. Energy giving food

1301. Term used for addition of nutrients to food that were not originally present.

A. Food enrichment

B. Food fortification

C. Food diversifiaction

D. None of these

1302. What is meant by enrichment in grain products?

A. Replacement of lost vitamins and minerals

B. Adding all minerals

C. Removal of vitamins and minerals

D. Adding all vitamins

1303. Which organisation carries out survey for determining the poverty line?

A. NSSO

B. CSO

C. Planning Commission

D. None of the above

1304. The calorie requirement is higher in the rural areas because:

A. They do not enjoy as much as people in the urban areas

B. Food items are expensive

C. They are engaged in mental work

D. People are engaged in physical labour

1305. The Food Safety and Standards Authority of India (FSSAI) has issued a set of guide-lines regarding the recall of _____ from the market.

A. Unsafe drinking water

B. Unsafe food products

C. Unsafe labeling

D. Unsafe packaging

1306. Which of the following is not a reason for increased risk of vitamin or mineral deficiencies among older people in high income countries?

A. Low income so decreased ability to purchase nutrient-rich foods

B. Decreased mobility and little time spend outdoors in the sunshine

C. Decreased intrinsic factor in the stomach

D. High nutrient requirements for tissue turnover

1307. Which is the good sources of protein?

A. Green vegetables B. Rice

C. Fruits D. Eggs

1308. Vitamin C or ascorbic acid yet another essential component of our diets. It keeps teeth, gums and joints healthy, and also holds cells together and increases our body's resistance to infection. A deficiency of vitamin C leads to bleeding and swollen gums, weight-loss, joint-pains, susceptibility to infection, and delayed wound-healing.

What is this condition called?

A. Scurvy

B. Goiter

C. Anemia

D. Marasmus

1309. Which one of the following is the correct sequence in the decreasing order of production (in million tonnes) of the given foodgrains in India?

A. Wheat – rice – pulses – coarse cereals

B. Rice – wheat – pulses – coarse cereals

C. Wheat – rice – coarse cereals – pulses

D. Rice – wheat – coarse cereals – pulses

1310. The eyes of potato are useful for:

A. Nutrition

B. Respiration

C. Vegetative propagation

D. Protection from predators

1311. Which of the following crops would be preferred for sowing in order to enrich the soil with nitrogen?

A. Wheat

B. Mustard

C. Sunflower

D. Gram

1312. Why is food safety important?

A. To prevent and stop food-borne illness and contaminants from getting into food and creating an outbreak

B. No loss of sales or business

C. To maintain a good reputation for the business

D. All of the above

1313. What is the function of vitamin K in our body?

A. Good vision

B. Smooth skin

C. Blood clotting

D. RBC formation

1314. This nutrient helps insulate our body and cushion our organs?

A. Water   B. Calcium

C. Potassium   D. Fat

1315. Which dietary component helps to maintain a constant body temperature in our body?

A. Roughage

B. Vitamins

C. Water

D. Energy giving food

1316. What is the name of the co-enzyme Q10?

A. Carenone

B. Ubiquinone

C. Quinone

D. None of above

1317. Omega 3 fatty acid is also known by what other name?

A. Olive oil

B. Linolenic acid

C. Fish oil

D. Lenoleic acid

1318. Full form of HFCS with reference to sweeteners?

A. High fructose corn syrup

B. High fat corn substitute

C. High frying corn substitute

D. None of the above

1319. Colustrum is very good as it is rich in:

A. Protein and carbohydrate

B. Proteins and antibodies

C. Minerals and vitamins

D. All of the above

1320. Weight gained per gram of protein consumed is known as:

A. BV   B. NPU

C. PER   D. NPR

1321. Of the microorganisms, _____ are the greatest threat to food safety.

A. Viruses

B. Fungi

C. Parasites

D. Bacteria

1322. Eradication of _____ is essential to improve access to food.

A. Malnutrition

B. Poverty

C. Undernutrition

D. Terrorism

1323. _____ functions in carbohydrate metabolism.

A. Zinc   B. Riboflavin

C. Thiamin   D. Vitamin B

1324. Fiber is important in ____ function.

A. Bowel

B. Muscle

C. Stomach

D. Skeletal

1325. Statement 1: Salt inhibits the heat resistance of bacteria.

Statement 2: Phosphate ions are important in spore formation.

A. True, false   B. True, true

C. False, false   D. False, true

1326. Isha noticed that fruits after ripening lived shorter than fresh vegetables. Which of the sentences pertaining to the above observation are correct?

A. Her observation was wrong

B. Fruits have old cells as they were not meant to be survived by nature

C. They can heal wounds

D. They can live longer

1327. Rinky learns how different minerals and vitamins are affected when exposed to certain conditions. Which one of them did she NOT comprehend properly?

A. When milk is exposed to sun, it losses vitamin B_2

B. Unless refrigerated immediately, meat losses vitamin C

C. Fats and oil in cold conditions, get spoilt

D. Microorganisms are a major threat to the food industry

1328. Which of the following is NOT a process wherein the food becomes toxin before ingestion?

A. Botulism

B. Staphylococcus

C. Bacterial intoxication

D. Bacterial infection

1329. Statement 1: Botulism is more dangerous than Staphylococcus.

Statement 2: Botulism is encountered by humans only if they have eaten the toxin. The organism in itself is no harm. Staphylococcus needs air and grows on warm food only.

A. True, false   B. True, true

C. False, false   D. False, true

1330. Statement 1: Processing contaminants are the contaminants that are generated during the processing of food and hence are hard to control.

Statement 2: Packaging materials also cause contamination.

A. True, false   B. True, true

C. False, false   D. False, true

1331. Statement 1: Certain new contaminants called emerging contaminants are contaminants which are a relatively new discovery.

Statement 2: Packaging materials should have sanitary precautions and agricultural products should be sterilized.

A. True, false   B. True, true

C. False, false   D. False, true

1332. The physical property that influences the deterioration of grain is _____

 A. Its flow properties

 B. Absorption, adsorption and desorption

 C. Porosity and its tendency towards layering

 D. All of the mentioned

1333. Statement 1: _____ packaging helps increase shelf-life of milk.

 Statement 2: Spoilage patterns for milk, eggs and meat are the same.

 A. Septic, false

 B. Aseptic, true

 C. Aseptic, false

 D. Septic, true

1334. Which information is incorrect when it comes to dehydration affecting vitamins?

 A. Beta-carotene and B-vitamin do not get affected

 B. Vitamin C does not get affected

 C. Vitamin C is retained during pickling of vegetables

 D. None of the mentioned

1335. Which of the following is untrue?

 A. Many vitamin Bs like vitamin B_6 are affected by heating

 B. Vitamin C is lost in almost all food processing steps

 C. Vitamin C degradation decreases by enzymes and also metals like Cu and Fe

 D. Vitamin A is stable in absence of oxygen

1336. Which of the following statements is true with respect to food processing?

 A. Sodium is lost during cooking and selenium is volatile and is lost by cooking or processing

 B. Vitamins can be removed from food via leaching

 C. Mineral losses in food processing are more compared to vitamins

 D. Boiling has less mineral losses as compared to steaming

1337. Which of the following operation reduces the dietary fibre content in cereals?

 A. Drying

 B. Retrogradation

 C. Grinding

 D. Milling

1338. Which of the following is a food safety tool?

 A. Good hygiene practice

 B. Hazard analysis critical control point

 C. Total quality management

 D. All of the mentioned

1339. Hazards affecting food are _____

 A. Chemical, biological, physical

 B. Additives, colour

 C. Pollutants

 D. All of the mentioned

1340. Which of the following terms refers to the amount of protein absorbed by the body from a food source?

 A. Biological value

 B. Limiting value

 C. Reference pattern

 D. None of the mentioned

1341. Which of the following is untrue?

 A. Biological value of plant sources is more than animal sources

 B. BV value of egg white is 100 that means almost the entire amount of nitrogen in egg white can be absorbed and used by the body

 C. Food energy is the amount of energy available from food through respiration

 D. Fats have the maximum amount of food energy

1342. Which of the following is untrue?

 A. Gut flora produces vitamin K and biotin in the intestine

 B. Vitamin D is synthesized in the skin

 C. Humans can produce some vitamins from precursors that they consume

 D. None of the mentioned

1343. Which of the following is false?

    A. Primary deficiency occurs when any vitamin is not consumed in the minimum required amount

    B. Secondary deficiency occurs when proper absorption of the vitamins does not take place

    C. Overdosing from vitamin supplementation is possible

    D. None of the mentioned

1344. Which one of the following mineral elements is required for muscle contraction?

    A. Calcium   B. Iron

    C. Sodium   D. Zinc

1345. Which of the following cannot be a part of a vegan diet?

    1. Eggs   2. Fish

    3. Milk   4. Vegetables

    A. 1 and 2

    B. 1, 2 and 3

    C. Only 2

    D. All of the above

1346. Which of the following is considered a complete protein food?

    A. Almond   B. Horse gram

    C. Soya bean   D. Cashew nut

1347. Which of the following nutrients is needed for a healthy immune system?

    A. Calcium   B. Iodine

    C. Vitamin K   D. Vitamin C

1348. Washing of peeled vegetables removes the vitamin?

    A. E   B. D

    C. C   D. B

1349. Statement 1: In microwave heating, heat is not applied to the food item.

Statement 2: Radiation does not gives even drying whereas microwave heating does.

    A. True, false   B. True, true

    C. False, false   D. False, true

1350. Which of the following information is required prior to launching a new product?

    A. Product and raw material specifications

    B. Process development

    C. Plant location and operation

    D. All of the mentioned

1351. Which of the following is not a function of a food additive?

    A. To maintain product consistency

    B. Maintain nutritive value

    C. Controlling acidity/alkalinity

    D. None of the mentioned

1352. Statement 1: Stabilizers, emulsifiers are certain examples of food additives.

Statement 2: Antioxidant is a class of food additive.

    A. True, false   B. True, true

    C. False, false   D. False, true

1353. Statement 1: In control of yeast in industries, baking soda is added (which is sodium bicarbonate) react with an acid which is externally added to release carbon dioxide which escapes?

Statement 2: Baking soda is a leavening agent. It is an additive.

    A. True, false   B. True, true

    C. False, false   D. False, true

1354. When food is given in the stomach or intestines directly then it is _____ nutrition.

    A. Intravenous   B. Saline

    C. Enteral   D. Parenteral

1355. To overcome diabetes, a person can increase the intake of _____ and reduce the intake of _____

    A. Carbohydrates, proteins

    B. Proteins, fats

    C. fats, carbohydrates

    D. Carbohydrates, fats

1356. For a person suffering from problems like slow neural transmission, e.g. dementia, they should be given _____
   A. Increased sodium
   B. Increased potassium
   C. Increased calcium
   D. Increased magnesium

1357. Which is an anti-hemorrhagic vitamin?
   A. Vitamin A   B. Vitamin K
   C. Vitamin E   D. Vitamin C

1358. Which is known as vinegar bacteria?
   A. *Lactobacillus*   B. *Acetobactor*
   C. *Clostridium*   D. *Bacillus*

1359. Solution of salt in water is called:
   A. Vinegar   B. Cider
   C. Juice   D. Brine

1360. The best evidence exists for which nutrients in the prevention of age related cognitive decline?
   A. N-3 fatty acids
   B. Phytochemicals
   C. N-6 fatty acids
   D. Long chain saturated fats

1361. Government scientists have calculated that a poor diet combined with a lack of sufficient physical activity accounts for 300,000 deaths due to heart disease, cancer and diabetes each year. Which of the following terms best describes this statement?
   A. Double blind   B. Risk factor
   C. Placebo   D. Chronic

1362. Carbohydrates, lipids, and proteins all contain carbon, hydrogen, and oxygen. Which one also contains nitrogen?
   A. Carbohydrates B. Lipids
   C. Proteins   D. Water

1363. A function of carbohydrates in the diet is to:
   A. Enable chemical reactions
   B. Promote growth and repair of tissues

   C. Suppy energy
   D. Maintain water balance

1364. Good sources of carbohydrate are:
   A. Fats, oils, butter, and margarine.
   B. Fish, eggs, beef, pork, and poultry
   C. Cereals, fruits, vegetables, and milk
   D. Green leafy vegetables, seafood, and water

1365. Functions of lipids in the diet are to:
   A. Provide fats essential for body function
   B. Transport water-soluble vitamins
   C. Promote growth and repair of tissue
   D. Maintain fluid balance

1366. Lipids are supplied in large quantities in the diet by:
   A. Fats, oils, meats, and nuts
   B. Cereals, fruits, vegetables, and breads
   C. Deep green and orange vegetables
   D. Green pepper, broccoli, cantaloupe, and citrus fruits.

1367. Essential nutrients:
   A. Are made by the body
   B. Generally must be supplied by food
   C. Include alcohol
   D. Are enzymes

1368. A kilocalorie (kcal) is a:
   A. Measure of fat weight
   B. Unit for expressing energy content in food
   C. Scientific instrument
   D. Term used to describe the amount of sugar and fat in food

1369. Which of the following is the term for substances that are both required by the body and that must be obtained from diet?
   A. Food
   B. Nutrients
   C. Essential foods
   D. Essential dietary needs

1370. Movement of food through much of the digestive system is done via which form of muscle action?

A. Peristalsis

B. Secretion

C. Sphincter contraction

D. Bolus segmentation

1371. A group of lactic acid producing bacteria that appear to provide a range of positive digestive benefits are known as:

A. Probiotics

B. Nutribiotics

C. Gastro-biotics

D. Bioproductives

1372. Gastroesophageal reflux disease (GERD) is a digestive disorder that:

A. Occurs when the valve at the top of the stomach relaxes

B. Occurs when the liver is in poor health

C. Is related to kidney functions

D. Is related to the presence of some heart condition

1373. The genetically-modified (GM) brinjal in India has been developed for:

A. Enhancing shelf life

B. Insect resistance

C. Drought resistance

D. Enhancing mineral content

1374. Sterilization of tissue culture medium is done by:

A. Mixing the medium with antifungal agents

B. Filtering the medium through fine sieve

C. Autoclaving of medium at 120° for 15 min

D. Keeping the medium at –20°C

1375. An improved variety of transgenic basmati rice

A. Gives high yield and is rich in vitamin A

B. Does not require chemical fertilizers and growth hormones

C. Give high yield but has no characteristic aroma

D. Is completely resistant to all insect pests and diseases of paddy

1376. Paste you _____ is a new-product development approach in which one company department works to complete its stage of the process before passing the new product along to the next department and stage.

A. Product life-cycle analysis

B. Sequential product development

C. Simultaneous product development

D. Team-based product development

1377. A detailed version of a new idea stated in meaningful customer terms is called a _____.

A. Product idea

B. Product movement

C. Product image

D. Product concept

1378. A manufacturer with a product in the decline stage of the product life cycle might decide to _____ if it has reason to hope that competitors will leave the industry.

A. Drop the product

B. Maintain the product without change

C. Search for replacements˙

D. Delay planning

1379. After concept testing, a firm would engage in which stage in developing and marketing a new product?

A. Test marketing

B. Product development

C. Marketing strategy development

D. Idea screening

1380. An attractive idea must be developed into a _____.

A. Product idea   B. Test market

C. Product concept   D. Product strategy

1381. During which stage of new-product development is management most likely to estimate minimum and maximum sales to assess the range of risk in launching a new product?
   A. Product development
   B. Marketing strategy development
   C. Test marketing
   D. Business analysis

1382. Executives, manufacturing employees, and salespeople are all examples of _____.
   A. Research and development team members
   B. Core members of innovation management systems
   C. Internal sources for new-product ideas
   D. External sources for new-product ideas

1383. In the _____ stage, the firm faces a trade-off between high market share and high current profit.
   A. Decline
   B. Growth
   C. Commercialization
   D. Introduction

1384. In the concept testing stage of new-product development, a product concept in _____ form is presented to groups of target consumers.
   A. Market tested
   B. Physical or symbolic
   C. Final
   D. Prototype

1385. Increasing profits will most likely occur at which stage of the PLC?
   A. Decline
   B. Introduction
   C. Growth
   D. Product development

1386. Most products in the marketplace are in the _____ stage of the product life cycle.
   A. Introduction
   B. Decline

C. Maturity
   D. Development

1387. Sales decline in the decline stage of the PLC because of technological advances, increased competition, and _____.
   A. Shifts in consumer tastes and preferences
   B. Shifts in the economy
   C. Marketing mix modifications
   D. Shifts in unemployment

1388. The major purpose of test marketing is to provide management with the information needed to make a final decision about _____.
   A. How to compete in the market
   B. How to develop a market strategy
   C. Which market to compete in
   D. Whether to launch the new product

1389. The PLC concept can be applied by marketers as a useful framework for describing how _____.
   A. Product ideas are developed
   B. To develop marketing strategies
   C. To forecast product performance
   D. Products and markets work

1390. The search for new-product ideas should be _____ rather than haphazard.
   A. Strategically planned
   B. Segmented
   C. Intermittent
   D. Systematic

1391. The team-based new-product development approach is faster because departments work closely together through _____.
   A. Cross-functional teams
   B. A step-by-step process
   C. Departmentalization
   D. Team efforts

1392. Under what circumstances might it be wise for a company to do little or no test marketing?

A. When management is not sure of the product

B. When the product has no substitutes and is new in its category

C. When management is not sure of the marketing program

D. When the costs of developing and introducing the product are low

1393. What are the two ways that a company can obtain new products?

A. Internal development and merger

B. New-product development and acquisition

C. Market mix modification and research and development

D. Line extension and brand management

1394. Which of the following cannot be described by the PLC concept?

A. Styles

B. Brand

C. Product form

D. Product image

1395. Which of the following costs is most likely associated with the commercialization stage of new-product development?

A. Determining the product's planned price, distribution, and marketing budget

B. Identifying target markets

C. Building or renting a manufacturing facility

D. Developing a prototype of the product

1396. Which of the following is not a potential cause of the failure of a new product?

A. A poorly designed product

B. An underestimated market size

C. Ineffective advertising

D. An incorrectly positioned product

1397. Which of the following is a disadvantage of a team-based approach to new-product development?

A. Levels of risk can be more easily controlled.

B. The process does not work with the shorter life cycles of many of today's products.

C. Organizational confusion and tension can be a part of the process.

D. It takes longer to get the right products to market.

1398. Which of the following is necessary for successful new-product development?

A. A market pioneer mindset and a holistic approach

B. A team-based, innovation-management approach

C. A holistic and sequential product development approach

D. A customer-centered, team-based, systematic approach

1399. Which of the following is perhaps the most important external source of new-product ideas?

A. Competitors

B. Customers

C. Trade magazines, shows, and seminars

D. Distributors and suppliers

1400. Which stage in the PLC normally lasts longer and poses strong challenges to the marketing managers?

A. Phase-in   B. Growth

C. Introduction   D. Maturity

1401. Your firm wants to use external sources for new product ideas. After consulting with a friend you learn that all of the following are common external sources except _____.

A. Customers

B. Trade shows and magazines

C. The firm's executives

D. Suppliers

1402. The fermentation process of producing black tea is an example of:
    A. Enzymatic fermentation
    B. Microbial fermentation
    C. Both A and B
    D. None of the above

1403. Who was the first zymologist and defined fermentations as "respiration without air"?
    A. Louis Pasteur
    B. Elie Metchinikoff
    C. Anthony Hopkins
    D. Emil Hansen

1404. Carbohydrate content in potato is:
    A. 12%   B. 22%
    C. 32%   D. 42%

1405. Which refrigerant is commonly us:
    A. Ethylene   B. Carbide
    C. Ammonia   D. Sodium benzoate

1406. Mango variety having strong flavour is:
    A. Dashart   B. Sindhu
    C. Langra   D. Fazli

1407. Which of the following is an advantage of food processing?
    A. Availability of seasonal food throughout the year
    B. Removal of toxins and preserving food for longer
    C. Adds extra nutrients to some food items
    D. All of the mentioned

1408. Which of the following is a disadvantage of food processing?
    A. Canning of food leads to loss of vitamin C
    B. Processed food adds empty calories to food constituting junk
    C. Some chemicals make the human and animal cells grow rapidly which is unhealthy
    D. All of the mentioned

1409. Which of the following is a performance parameter for the food industry?
    A. Hygiene
    B. Labour used
    C. Hygiene and labour used
    D. None of the above

1410. Statement 1: Cost reduction trend of the food industry often leads manufacturers to forget the health aspect of the food, although health itself is another important trend of the food industry.

    Statement 2: Food processing industry nowadays is also looking into energy efficiency methods to process food. Hence it is an upcoming trend.
    A. True, false
    B. True, true
    C. False, false
    D. False, true

1411. Which of the following parts of a plant are spices not made from?
    A. Bark
    B. Leaf
    C. Root
    D. Cell

1412. The Queen of spices is _____
    A. Cardamom
    B. Pepper
    C. Ginger
    D. Chilly

1413. Statement 1: Black pepper is obtained from ripened berries by removing the pulp.

    Statement 2: White pepper is obtained by plucking a few cherries which have turned orange/red, are spread on the floor and are separated by trampling.
    A. True, false
    B. True, true
    C. False, false
    D. False, true

1414. Statement 1: Chillies are pungent in nature.

Statement 2: Chillies are pungent due to the presence of the compound capsaicin.

A. True, false   B. True, true

C. False, false   D. False, true

1415. Which of the following is untrue about ginger?

A. It is a rhizome

B. Scraping the outer skin of ginger needs to be taken care of because if the essential oils are stripped off, ginger loses its aroma

C. All of the mentioned

D. None of the mentioned

1416. Which of the following is true about turmeric?

A. Green rhizomes are boiled in water till a froth comes out and white fumes appear giving out a characteristic odour

B. The softness of the cooked rhizomes depends on the curing conditions and process.

C. After drying, the turmeric hardens up

D. All of the mentioned

1417. The aromatic volatile components of spices are called _____

A. Spice oil   B. Spice fat

C. Spice gel   D. Spice paste

1418. Which one of the following bacteria causes the greatest number of cases of food poisoning?

A. *Clostridium perfringens*

B. *Listeria*

C. *Staphylococcus aureus*

D. *Salmonella*

1419. The main symptom of *Staphylococcus* food poisoning is:

A. Vomiting   B. Diarrhea

C. Fever   D. Abdominal pains

1420. Which of the following statements are true?

A. Pectin is a reversible colloid

B. Addition of sugar influences the pectin water equilibrium

C. With the increase in acidity, the pectin structure fibers are tougher

D. All of the mentioned

1421. Why is powdered pectin mixed ten times with its volume in dry sugar, mixed thoroughly and added to the juice?

A. It gives a better taste

B. To solidify the juice to form jelly

C. Uniform distribution and prevent lumping

D. All of the mentioned

1422. Which of the following is true about jellies?

A. If acid needs to be added to compensate for the deficiencies in fruit composition, it is best added at the end of the evaporation cycle

B. Addition of acid late to the jelly allows formation of it in the container before gel formation

C. Setting of jelly can be controlled by part by the addition of sodium citrate

D. All of the above

1423. Which of the following is not a step in modern milling of wheat?

A. Stone grinding

B. Wheat conditioning

C. Wheat milling

D. Cleaning

1424. Which of the following is not a part of a wheat kernel?

A. Bran

B. Endosperm

C. Germ

D. None of the above

1425. Which of the following statements is false?

A. Rice can be milled by a solvent method in which the solvent softens the bran layer of the rice

B. Advantage of the solvent process is that it has lesser fat content

C. Lesser fat content increases the shelf life of the rice

D. None of the above

1426. Which one of the following food item does not provide dietary fibre?

A. Whole grains

B. Whole pulses

C. Fruits and vegetables

D. Milk

1427. Which of the following sources of protein is different from others?

A. Peas

B. Gram

C. Soya bean

D. Cottage cheese (paneer)

1428. Which of the following nutrients is not present in milk?

A. Protein

B. Vitamin C

C. Calcium

D. Vitamin D

1429. Read the food items given below:

i. Wheat

ii. Ghee

iii. Iodised salt

iv. Spinach (palak)

Which of the above food items are "energy giving foods"?

A. (i) and (iv)

B. (ii) and (iv)

C. (i) and (ii)

D. (iii) and (iv)

1430. Read the following statements about diseases.

i. They are caused by germs.

ii. They are caused due to lack of nutrients in our diet.

iii. They can be passed onto another person through contact.

iv. They can be prevented by taking a balanced diet.

Which pair of statements best describe a deficiency disease?

A. (i) and (ii)

B. (ii) and (iii)

C. (ii) and (iv)

D. (i) and (iii)

1431. Given below are the steps to test the presence of proteins in a food item:

i. Take a small quantity of the food item in a test tube, add 10 drops of water to it and shake it.

ii. Make a paste or powder of food to be tested.

iii. Add 10 drops of caustic soda solution to the test tube and shake well.

iv. Add 2 drops of copper sulphate solution to it.

Which of the following is the correct sequence of the steps?

A. i, ii, iv, iii

B. ii, i, iv, iii

C. ii, i, iii, iv

D. iv, ii, i, iii

1432. Fruits, vegetables and cereals are potent sources of:

A. Antioxidants   B. Unsaturated fat

C. Saturated fat   D. Free radicals

1433. The leading source of antioxidants in the diet is:

A. Citrus fruits   B. Spinach

C. Coffee   D. Egg yolks

1434. The essential fatty acids that must be derived from the diet are:

A. Stearidonic acid and eicosatetraenoic acid

B. Eicosapentaenoic acid and docosapentaenoic acid

C. Linoleic and alpha-linoleic acid

D. Gamma-linoleic acid and arachidonic acid

1435. All of the following statements about omega-3 fatty acids are true *except:*

A. They help to maintain healthy triglyceride and high-density lipoprotein

B. They have significantly contributed to the obesity epidemic

C. They are necessary for healthy infant growth and development

D. They play an important role in the production of hormones that govern numerous metabolic and biological processes

1436. All of the following may be associated with scurvy *except:*

A. Loss of appetite and irritability

B. Diarrhea and fever

C. Tenderness and swelling in legs

D. First symptom is altered mental status

1437. The only fat-soluble antioxidant synthesized in the body is:

A. Vitamin D   B. Thiamine

C. Ascorbic acid   D. CoQ10

1438. Good source of vitamin D include all *except:*

A. Blueberries

B. Sunlight

C. Salmon, tuna sardines and mackerel

D. Fortified milk and other dairy products

1439. One of the fat-soluble vitamins involved in coagulation is:

A. Vitamin K   B. Vitamin A

C. Vitamin D   D. Vitamin E

1440. Products that contain live microorganisms in sufficient numbers to alter intestinal microflora and promote intestinal microbial balance are known as:

A. Antibiotics

B. Probiotics

C. Fruits and vegetables

D. Digestive enzymes

1441. Nondigestible food ingredients that stimulate the growth and activity of certain bacteria in the colon are called:

A. Insoluble fiber   B. Probiotics

C. Prebiotics   D. Cellulose

1442. A deficiency of thiamine (vitamin B_1) in the diet causes:

A. Osteopenia

B. Beriberi

C. Protein malnutrition

D. Scurvy

1443. All of the following statements about vitamin B_3 (niacin) are true *except:*

A. It helps to release energy in carbohydrates, fat, and protein

B. It improves blood lipid levels

C. Deficiency causes beriberi

D. It is involved in the synthesis of sex hormones

1444. All of the following are potentially modifiable risk factors for osteoporosis *except:*

A. Anorexia nervosa

B. Chronically low intake of calcium and vitamin D

C. Chronically low intake of vitamins C and B_6

D. Excessive alcohol consumption

1445. Characteristics of successful dieters include all of the following *except:*

A. Maintaining a daily food journal

B. Counting calories

C. Adhering to a strict eating plan

D. Eliminating all carbohydrates from their diets

1446. Iron supplements are frequently recommended for all of the following *except:*
A. Women who are pregnant
B. Infants and toddlers
C. Teenage girls
D. Postmenopausal women

1447. Which of the following is a factor that affects the storage stability of food?
A. Type of raw material used
B. Quality of raw material used
C. Method/effectiveness of packaging
D. All of the mentioned

1448. Which of the following sentences is true with respect to food storage/preservation?
A. Each food type has a potential storage life
B. The mechanical abuse that food has received during storage/distribution does not affects its storage stability
C. All of the mentioned
D. None of the mentioned

1449. Choose the true statement.
A. Food storage and preservation is observed to be better/easier in parts of the world that have civilizations prevalent there
B. Proteins are held in an emulsion state in a water system
C. Fats are in colloidal state
D. All of the above

1450. Which of the following statement with respect to food preservation is true?
A. Leafy vegetables perish fast due to their high moisture content
B. Cereals have the highest requirements of moisture and soil types
C. Cereal can be grown with less labour and yield of food is high
D. All of the above

1451. What benefits are there in eating a balanced diet?
A. Good health
B. Good mood and energy
C. Improved health and reduced illness
D. All of the above.

1453. Which of the following is a macronutrient?
A. Vitamin A   B. Selenium
C. Protein   D. Antioxidants

1454. Which of the following provides the body with zero calories per gram?
A. Carbohydrates   B. Protein
C. Lipids   D. Water

1455. When scientists use the word "calorie", what are they referring to?
A. One gram of fat
B. One gram of carbohydrates
C. Enough energy to raise the temperature of one gram of water by 1°C
D. 10 grams of fat

1456. Which of the following is not an example of a carbohydrate?
A. Starch   B. Sucrose
C. Glycogen   D. Cholesterol

1457. What defines all carbohydrates?
A. They all have the formula $(CH_2O)n$
B. They all contain carbon, hydrogen and only one oxygen
C. They all contain oxygen and nitrogen
D. They are all made of long chains of sugars

1458. Which of the following is a carbohydrate, AND is found in large quantities in a potato?
A. Starch
B. Pure glucose
C. Pure fructose
D. Stearic acid

1459. Which of the following is NOT a function of polysaccharides in human nutrition?
   A. Energy
   B. Fiber
   C. Prevents ketoacidosis
   D. Building enzymes

1460. Which form of carbohydrate does the human body use to store energy?
   A. Starch   B. Cellulose
   C. Glycogen   D. Chitin

1461. Which of the following is not a function of protein?
   A. Provides several important players in the immune system
   B. Acid–base balance
   C. Muscular contraction
   D. Protein is the body's first choice for an energy source.

1462. When do we expect to see positive nitrogen balance?
   A. When the body is building itself back up after an illness
   B. When the body is being broken down by an illness
   C. During starvation
   D. When we eat a lot of protein

1463. The negative logarithm of the molar concentration of H+ ions in aqueous solutions is called:
   A. Self-ionization of water
   B. Hydrogenation
   C. pH
   D. Equilibrium constant

1465. Phytochemicals are _____.
   A. Nutrients that do not provide health benefits
   B. Available only as supplements
   C. Required in the diet
   D. Active compounds that are found in plants

1466. Free radicals, a type of pro-oxidant, _____.
   A. Are a type of phytochemical
   B. Increase the risk of cardiovascular disease
   C. Are a type of non-phytochemical
   D. Were part of the 1960s anti-war movement

1467. Which of these antioxidants, when taken in excess, may promote oxidation?
   A. Vitamins J and M
   B. Zinc and oxygen
   C. Beta-carotene, and vitamins C and E
   D. Selenium, calcium and thiamin

1468. Which of the following dietary patterns has a positive correlation with markers of inflammation?
   A. One that emphasizes whole grains over refined grains
   B. Mediterranean
   C. Vegetable-rich
   D. Red-meat based

1469. Moderate coffee consumption may decrease the risk of all of the following except _____.
   A. Osteoporosis   B. Dementia
   C. Type 2 diabetes   D. Liver cancer

1470. When consumed from foods, beta-carotene is a(n) _____.
   A. Free radical
   B. Poison
   C. Antioxidant
   D. Dangerous to the human body

1471. Beta-carotene supplements, if taken by a smoker, may _____.
   A. Decrease the risk of cardiovascular disease
   B. Increase the risk of death
   C. Increase the risk of gout
   D. Decrease the risk of lung cancer

1472. The primary function of vitamin E is as a(n) _____.

A. Component of insulin

B. Hormone

C. Promoter of mineral absorption

D. Antioxidant

1473. Vitamin E is relatively non-toxic, however, excessive intake may _____.

A. Promote vitamin K activity

B. Interfere with the absorption of minerals

C. Interfere with blood clotting

D. Interfere with the absoption of vitamin A

1474. Many phytochemicals (active compounds found in plants) promote health by _____.

A. Raising LDL cholestrol

B. Acting as an anti-inflammatory

C. Lowering HDL

D. Promoting oxidation

1475. Which of the following contains the most resveratrol—an antioxidant and anti-inflammatory compound? (Resveratrol is a type of natural phenol produced by several plants in response to injury) Hint: The skin of blueberries, raspberries, and grapes are great sources.

A. Red roses   B. Red potatoes

C. Red wine   D. Red meat

1476. Organosulfur compounds (organic compounds that contain sulfur) are antioxidant, anticancer, and antimicrobial compounds. Which of the following is especially rich in organosulfur compounds?

A. Beets   B. Carrot

C. Oranges   D. Garlic

1477. Which of the following is rich in vitamin E?

A. Nuts   B. Squash

C. Pears   D. Apples

1478. This is for all you coffee lovers! Which of the following coffee preparation methods is best for health?

A. Light roast and paper filter

B. Dark roast expresso

C. Dark roast and french press

D. Light roast and boil the grounds

1479. True tea comes from only one source: *Camellia sinensis*—a species of small tree or evergreen shrub. Which of the following is true about the consumption of true tea (not herbal tea)?

A. Reduces the risk of cancer

B. Increases LDL

C. Decreases HDL

D. Reduces risk of osteoporosis

1480. Vitamin C reduces the formation of nitrosamines in the stomach. What are nitrosamines?

A. Carcinogens (a substance capable of causing cancer in living tissue)

B. Inhibitors of calcium absorption

C. Blood cells

D. Fruits and vegetables

1481. In your body, carotenoids (a class of mainly orange, yellow or red fat-soluble pigments which give color to plants) especially beta-carotene, can be converted into _____.

A. Iron

B. Vitamin A

C. Vitamin E

D. Vitamin B_{12}

1482. If you want to reduce your risk of dementia, consume _____.

A. Butter

B. Blueberries

C. Poultry

D. Red meats

1483. Pro-oxidants are chemicals that induce oxidative stress. Which of the following does not result in the formation of pro-oxidants?

A. ATP (adenosine tri-phospate) production

B. Use of, and exposure to tobacco

C. C - exposure to UV radiation

D. All of the choices

1484. Polyphenols, found in foods such as citrus fruits, apples, tea, and blueberries, _____.

A. Reduce the risk of osteoporosis

B. Cure headaches instantly

C. Reduce inflammation

D. Heal bruises in one day

1485. A "nonself" substance that can provoke an immune response is called a(n) _____.

A. Immunoglobulin

B. Antibody

C. Colony-stimulating factor

D. Antigen

1486. Which of the following is true for single cell protein?

A. Algae cannot be used in single cell protein

B. It is produced through fermentation

C. It does not contain carbohydrates and vitamins

D. Its utilization increases environmental pollution

1487. Role of biotechnology in the production of food based on _____?

A. Decomposition   B. Respiration

C. Digestion   D. Fermentation

1488. Enzymes degrade, alter or synthesize a food component through:

A. Oxidation/reduction/isomerization

B. Hydrolysis/synthesis

C. Group transfer

D. All of the above

1489. Milk digestibility is improved by using:

A. RNase   B. Lactase

C. β-amylase   D. None of these

1490. Which of the following enzyme is responsible for causing vitamin B deficiency disease beriberi:

A. Ascorbic acid oxidase

B. Thiaminase

C. Lipoxygenase

D. None of these

1491. Health benefits of nutraceuticals are as follows:

A. They do not have any side effects

B. They have beneficial effect on health

C. Improves health

D. All of the above

1492. Water excretion is regulated by the brain and the:

A. Kidneys   B. Bloodstream

C. Stomach   D. Salivary glands

1493. Which among the following are not used as raw materials for alcohol production?

A. Corn   B. Molasses

C. Whey   D. Grapes

1494. Which of the following microorganism have high vitamin content?

A. Bacteria   B. Yeast

C. Algae   D. Protozoa

1495. A large group of people experience acute gastroenteritis 4–6 hours after eating custard pie. Which bacterium is most likely the culprit?

A. *Campylobacter jejuni*

B. *Listeria monocytogenes*

C. *Staphylococcus aureus*

D. *Vibrio parahaemolyticus*

1496. Which of the following is the primary cause of food-borne i!!ness?

A. Bacteria   B. Parasites

C. Protozoa   D. Viruses

1497. A high concentration of high density lipoproteins (HDLs) is associated with a:
A. High incidence of heart disease
B. High rate of nerve impulse transfer
C. Low incidence of heart disease
D. Low rate of nerve impulse

1498. *Acetobacor aceti* converts _____ into acetic acids
A. Ethyl alcohol
B. Glucose
C. Methyl alcohol
D. Starch

1499. What is fortification of food?
A. Deliberately increasing the content of an essential micronutrient in food
B. Providing tablets containing vitamins and minerals along with food
C. Proper cooking and storage of food to avoid loss of nutrient
D. Ensuring minimum amount of nutrients in food

1500. Any change that renders food unfit for human consumption is called:
A. Processing   B. Spoilage
C. Deterioration   D. Preservation

Answers

1. C	44. A	87. B	130. B	173. D	216. C	259. D	302. D	345. C	388. A
2. D	45. C	88. D	131. C	174. A	217. B	260. A	303. C	346. D	389. B
3. C	46. C	89. C	132. B	175. B	218. A	261. B	304. A	347. A	390. A
4. B	47. C	90. B	133. A	176. B	219. A	262. B	305. C	348. A	391. C
5. C	48. B	91. A	134. A	177. B	220. C	263. B	306. D	349. B	392. B
6. A	49. B	92. A	135. B	178. C	221. B	264. D	307. A	350. B	393. B
7. D	50. C	93. B	136. D	179. A	222. D	265. C	308. A	351. A	394. C
8. D	51. C	94. D	137. B	180. B	223. C	266. D	309. C	352. B	395. D
9. C	52. B	95. C	138. A	181. A	224. C	267. B	310. C	353. B	396. D
10. D	53. A	96. A	139. A	182. B	225. D	268. B	311. B	354. B	397. D
11. D	54. C	97. D	140. D	183. C	226. B	269. A	312. D	355. A	398. B
12. B	55. C	98. A	141. C	184. D	227. A	270. C	313. C	356. C	399. A
13. B	56. B	99. C	142. A	185. D	228. D	271. D	314. B	357. A	400. D
14. A	57. C	100. A	143. D	186. C	229. A	272. C	315. C	358. A	401. B
15. D	58. B	101. C	144. C	187. D	230. D	273. B	316. D	359. D	402. D
16. A	59. C	102. A	145. B	188. D	231. D	274. C	317. A	360. D	403. D
17. B	60. A	103. A	146. C	189. A	232. A	275. C	318. D	361. C	404. B
18. A	61. D	104. B	147. B	190. C	233. D	276. A	319. D	362. C	405. D
19. A	62. A	105. C	148. C	191. D	234. B	277. C	320. C	363. A	406. D
20. A	63. A	106. B	149. A	192. A	235. C	278. C	321. D	364. C	407. A
21. D	64. A	107. D	150. B	193. B	236. A	279. B	322. B	365. C	408. B
22. B	65. A	108. A	151. A	194. C	237. D	280. A	323. A	366. A	409. D
23. C	66. B	109. C	152. A	195. A	238. A	281. D	324. B	367. B	410. D
24. A	67. C	110. B	153. A	196. B	239. C	282. B	325. A	368. B	411. C
25. C	68. D	111. A	154. B	197. D	240. D	283. D	326. B	369. B	412. C
26. C	69. B	112. D	155. D	198. D	241. B	284. B	327. A	370. A	413. A
27. B	70. B	113. D	156. C	199. C	242. C	285. B	328. C	371. C	414. B
28. C	71. B	114. D	157. C	200. D	243. C	286. B	329. A	372. D	415. B
29. C	72. D	115. C	158. A	201. B	244. B	287. D	330. A	373. C	416. C
30. C	73. B	116. B	159. C	202. C	245. A	288. D	331. A	374. B	417. C
31. B	74. D	117. C	160. D	203. B	246. D	289. D	332. B	375. C	418. A
32. B	75. C	118. A	161. A	204. A	247. A	290. A	333. A	376. D	419. C
33. C	76. D	119. A	162. C	205. D	248. D	291. D	334. A	377. A	420. D
34. A	77. A	120. A	163. B	206. A	249. D	292. B	335. C	378. C	421. D
35. C	78. B	121. B	164. A	207. C	250. C	293. D	336. B	379. C	422. C
36. D	79. B	122. C	165. B	208. A	251. B	294. B	337. A	380. D	423. B
37. D	80. A	123. B	166. D	209. C	252. B	295. A	338. C	381. A	424. B
38. B	81. B	124. B	167. D	210. D	253. A	296. A	339. D	382. D	425. D
39. A	82. D	125. B	168. D	211. B	254. C	297. D	340. C	383. A	426. B
40. B	83. D	126. A	169. B	212. A	255. A	298. D	341. A	384. C	427. A
41. D	84. B	127. A	170. A	213. C	256. A	299. B	342. B	385. C	428. B
42. B	85. A	128. B	171. B	214. B	257. C	300. B	343. C	386. C	429. D
43. D	86. A	129. C	172. A	215. C	258. A	301. C	344. A	387. C	430. B

431. A	478. B	525. D	572. A	619. D	666. C	713. B	760. C	807. D	854. D
432. B	479. A	526. A	573. C	620. D	667. C	714. A	761. C	808. B	855. A
433. C	480. B	527. A	574. A	621. C	668. B	715. C	762. C	809. B	856. C
434. D	481. A	528. A	575. C	622. D	669. D	716. C	763. C	810. C	857. B
435. A	482. B	529. D	576. A	623. C	670. B	717. B	764. C	811. C	858. D
436. B	483. A	530. C	577. D	624. C	671. D	718. A	765. B	812. A	859. A
437. C	484. D	531. A	578. B	625. C	672. D	719. D	766. D	813. A	860. D
438. D	485. A	532. B	579. C	626. D	673. C	720. A	767. D	814. A	861. D
439. A	486. B	533. C	580. A	627. C	674. A	721. B	768. B	815. C	862. B
440. D	487. B	534. A	581. C	628. A	675. C	722. A	769. B	816. D	863. C
441. A	488. B	535. B	582. A	629. D	676. C	723. D	770. B	817. A	864. C
442. D	489. C	536. C	583. A	630. D	677. D	724. C	771. B	818. B	865. D
443. C	490. D	537. B	584. C	631. B	678. B	725. D	772. A	819. B	866. A
444. B	491. B	538. D	585. D	632. D	679. C	726. A	773. A	820. B	867. B
445. D	492. A	539. B	586. A	633. D	680. A	727. D	774. A	821. D	868. A
446. B	493. A	540. B	587. A	634. C	681. D	728. A	775. A	822. B	869. D
447. A	494. B	541. B	588. C	635. D	682. D	729. D	776. A	823. D	870. B
448. C	495. C	542. D	589. B	636. B	683. D	730. D	777. B	824. D	871. D
449. C	496. A	543. A	590. A	637. D	684. D	731. D	778. C	825. C	872. C
450. A	497. C	544. B	591. A	638. A	685. D	732. A	779. B	826. C	873. B
451. A	498. B	545. C	592. A	639. A	686. D	733. A	780. D	827. A	874. B
452. C	499. C	546. A	593. A	640. A	687. A	734. D	781. A	828. A	875. A
453. B	500. A	547. A	594. A	641. D	688. C	735. D	782. C	829. B	876. A
454. C	501. C	548. D	595. A	642. C	689. A	736. B	783. A	830. C	877. C
455. B	502. C	549. B	596. B	643. B	690. B	737. D	784. B	831. B	878. D
456. A	503. B	550. C	597. D	644. A	691. B	738. B	785. B	832. B	879. B
457. C	504. C	551. A	598. D	645. A	692. B	739. D	786. C	833. C	880. B
458. A	505. D	552. B	599. D	646. A	693. A	740. D	787. D	834. D	881. D
459. B	506. C	553. B	600. D	647. B	694. B	741. B	788. A	835. A	882. D
460. B	507. D	554. C	601. D	648. C	695. C	742. C	789. A	836. A	883. B
461. D	508. C	555. A	602. C	649. C	696. B	743. B	790. A	837. D	884. B
462. A	509. B	556. A	603. D	650. A	697. B	744. C	791. C	838. D	885. D
463. D	510. A	557. B	604. C	651. A	698. C	745. B	792. D	839. B	886. D
464. A	511. D	558. A	605. D	652. A	699. D	746. C	793. D	840. C	887. D
465. C	512. D	559. A	606. D	653. B	700. D	747. B	794. D	841. A	888. C
466. C	513. D	560. D	607. C	654. A	701. A	748. A	795. C	842. B	889. A
467. D	514. D	561. B	608. D	655. A	702. D	749. C	796. D	843. C	890. D
468. C	515. D	562. C	609. A	656. B	703. A	750. D	797. B	844. C	891. B
469. D	516. A	563. B	610. B	657. D	704. D	751. B	798. B	845. D	892. D
470. B	517. A	564. D	611. C	658. A	705. A	752. B	799. B	846. D	893. D
471. B	518. C	565. C	612. D	659. B	706. D	753. B	800. C	847. D	894. A
472. D	519. D	566. B	613. C	660. B	707. A	754. A	801. B	848. C	895. D
473. C	520. B	567. C	614. C	661. B	708. B	755. B	802. B	849. D	896. D
474. D	521. B	568. C	615. A	662. D	709. A	756. B	803. B	850. B	897. B
475. A	522. D	569. A	616. D	663. D	710. A	757. C	804. B	851. C	898. C
476. C	523. C	570. C	617. D	664. B	711. D	758. B	805. D	852. D	899. A
477. B	524. B	571. C	618. A	665. C	712. B	759. C	806. B	853. A	900. D

901. C	948. A	995. C	1042. A	1089. B	1136. A	1183. A	1230. D	1277. B	1324. A
902. D	949. D	996. B	1043. A	1090. A	1137. A	1184. D	1231. D	1278. D	1325. B
903. B	950. B	997. A	1044. B	1091. A	1138. D	1185. D	1232. D	1279. D	1326. C
904. C	951. B	998. B	1045. A	1092. D	1139. D	1186. D	1233. D	1280. D	1327. D
905. C	952. B	999. A	1046. D	1093. C	1140. D	1187. D	1234. B	1281. A	1328. B
906. C	953. A	1000. C	1047. B	1094. D	1141. D	1188. A	1235. B	1282. A	1329. B
907. A	954. C	1001. A	1048. B	1095. C	1142. C	1189. D	1236. C	1283. D	1330. B
908. B	955. B	1002. D	1049. D	1096. C	1143. A	1190. A	1237. D	1284. A	1331. B
909. C	956. D	1003. B	1050. B	1097. B	1144. B	1191. B	1238. D	1285. D	1332. D
910. D	957. B	1004. B	1051. C	1098. D	1145. C	1192. A	1239. A	1286. B	1333. B
911. A	958. C	1005. D	1052. A	1099. A	1146. A	1193. A	1240. D	1287. B	1334. C
912. C	959. D	1006. B	1053. B	1100. D	1147. C	1194. A	1241. B	1288. C	1335. C
913. B	960. A	1007. D	1054. D	1101. A	1148. B	1195. D	1242. B	1289. B	1336. A
914. D	961. A	1008. C	1055. C	1102. C	1149. C	1196. B	1243. A	1290. C	1337. D
915. A	962. D	1009. A	1056. A	1103. A	1150. B	1197. D	1244. C	1291. B	1338. D
916. C	963. B	1010. D	1057. B	1104. B	1151. A	1198. A	1245. B	1292. B	1339. D
917. B	964. A	1011. B	1058. A	1105. C	1152. D	1199. D	1246. C	1293. C	1340. A
918. A	965. A	1012. C	1059. C	1106. D	1153. D	1200. D	1247. B	1294. A	1341. A
919. D	966. A	1013. A	1060. B	1107. D	1154. B	1201. C	1248. D	1295. D	1342. D
920. B	967. D	1014. D	1061. A	1108. A	1155. D	1202. A	1249. B	1296. A	1343. A
921. A	968. D	1015. D	1062. D	1109. C	1156. B	1203. D	1250. D	1297. A	1344. A
922. D	969. C	1016. D	1063. D	1110. B	1157. D	1204. B	1251. B	1298. A	1345. B
923. C	970. D	1017. A	1064. D	1111. C	1158. A	1205. B	1252. A	1299. A	1346. D
924. B	971. B	1018. C	1065. C	1112. C	1159. B	1206. D	1253. A	1300. C	1347. D
925. B	972. A	1019. A	1066. A	1113. C	1160. D	1207. C	1254. D	1301. A	1348. C
926. D	973. B	1020. A	1067. A	1114. D	1161. A	1208. A	1255. C	1302. A	1349. B
927. A	974. B	1021. C	1068. B	1115. C	1162. D	1209. D	1256. D	1303. A	1350. D
928. A	975. D	1022. A	1069. A	1116. D	1163. D	1210. B	1257. A	1304. D	1351. D
929. D	976. D	1023. D	1070. D	1117. A	1164. C	1211. B	1258. B	1305. B	1352. B
930. C	977. D	1024. C	1071. A	1118. B	1165. B	1212. A	1259. C	1306. D	1353. B
931. B	978. A	1025. D	1072. C	1119. A	1166. C	1213. B	1260. B	1307. D	1354. C
932. C	979. C	1026. A	1073. B	1120. C	1167. D	1214. D	1261. A	1308. C	1355. B
933. C	980. D	1027. C	1074. B	1121. A	1168. B	1215. A	1262. B	1309. D	1356. B
934. B	981. C	1028. A	1075. D	1122. C	1169. A	1216. A	1263. C	1310. C	1357. B
935. C	982. D	1029. D	1076. A	1123. A	1170. B	1217. B	1264. C	1311. D	1358. B
936. B	983. A	1030. D	1077. B	1124. D	1171. C	1218. C	1265. D	1312. D	1359. D
937. B	984. A	1031. A	1078. C	1125. B	1172. B	1219. C	1266. D	1313. C	1360. A
938. C	985. B	1032. D	1079. D	1126. A	1173. A	1220. D	1267. C	1314. D	1361. B
939. B	986. A	1033. B	1080. B	1127. D	1174. A	1221. B	1268. A	1315. C	1362. B
940. A	987. C	1034. A	1081. C	1128. D	1175. D	1222. D	1269. D	1316. B	1363. C
941. B	988. A	1035. A	1082. C	1129. D	1176. C	1223. D	1270. B	1317. B	1364. C
942. A	989. A	1036. C	1083. D	1130. C	1177. A	1224. D	1271. D	1318. A	1365. A
943. C	990. D	1037. C	1084. C	1131. C	1178. C	1225. B	1272. A	1319. B	1366. A
944. B	991. B	1038. B	1085. C	1132. D	1179. D	1226. D	1273. B	1320. D	1367. B
945. C	992. D	1039. B	1086. A	1133. C	1180. A	1227. D	1274. C	1321. D	1368. B
946. A	993. A	1040. D	1087. B	1134. B	1181. A	1228. C	1275. D	1322. C	1369. B
947. C	994. B	1041. D	1088. D	1135. D	1182. A	1229. D	1276. B	1323. B	1370. A

1371. A	1384. B	1397. C	1410. D	1423. A	1436. D	1449. A	1462. A	1475. C	1488. B
1372. B	1385. C	1398. D	1411. A	1424. D	1437. D	1450. D	1463. C	1476. D	1489. B
1373. B	1386. C	1399. B	1412. C	1425. D	1438. D	1451. D	1464. D	1477. A	1490. B
1374. C	1387. A	1400. D	1413. B	1426. D	1439. A	1452. D	1465. B	1478. A	1491. D
1375. A	1388. D	1401. C	1414. B	1427. D	1440. B	1453. C	1466. C	1479. A	1492. A
1376. B	1389. D	1402. A	1415. D	1428. B	1441. C	1454. D	1467. C	1480. A	1493. C
1377. D	1390. D	1403. A	1416. D	1429. C	1442. B	1455. C	1468. D	1481. B	1494. C
1378. B	1391. A	1404. A	1417. A	1430. C	1443. C	1456. D	1469. A	1482. B	1495. C
1379. C	1392. D	1405. B	1418. D	1431. B	1444. C	1457. A	1470. C	1483. D	1496. A
1380. C	1393. B	1406. C	1419. A	1432. A	1445. D	1458. A	1471. B	1484. C	1497. C
1381. D	1394. D	1407. D	1420. D	1433. C	1446. D	1459. D	1472. D	1485. D	1498. A
1382. C	1395. C	1408. D	1421. C	1434. C	1447. D	1460. C	1473. C	1486. B	1499. A
1383. B	1396. B	1409. B	1422. D	1435. B	1448. A	1461. D	1474. B	1487. D	1500. B

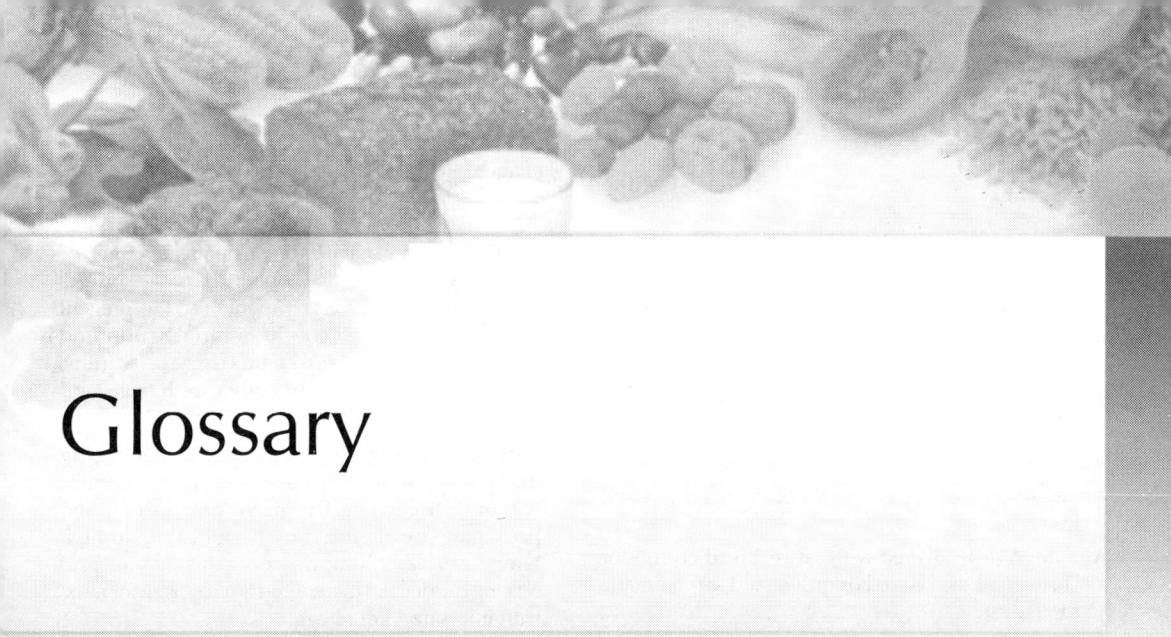

Glossary

A

Abrasion: An abrasion or "excoriation" is a wearing away of the upper layer of skin as a result of applied friction force. In dentistry an "abrasion" is the wearing away of the tooth substance.

Absorption: The amount of water flour can take up and hold while being made into simple dough. Absorption is based on predetermined standard dough consistency or stiffness; expressed as a percentage of weight of flour.

Acceptable daily intake (ADI): Quantity of a food additive that can be ingested daily, over a lifetime, without any risk (expressed in milligrams additive per kilogram body weight).

Acetic acid: A simple organic acid used for preserving foods.

Acid: Sour-tasting compound containing hydrogen that may be ionized or replaced by positive elements to form salts.

Acrolein: Irritating substance formed by the decomposition of glycerol at high temperatures.

Active packaging: Contains active component allowing a controlled interaction between the food, package and internal gaseous environment, thus extends shelf life, improves fruit and vegetable safety or provides superior sensory quality.

Adapt: Aler to suit the new condition or use.

Additives: Additives are substances added to food, to preserve or enhance flavors or appearance.

Adrenaline: A hormone secreted by the body in response to stress.

Adulteration: The addition or contamination of a food by a substance foreign to the normal product, which debases it or disguises inferior quality.

Aerobic: Requiring oxygen to live and grow; said of some bacteria.

Aflatoxins: A powerful mycotoxin produced by the Aspergeillus mold, which is a ssociation with crops such as peanuts, corn, rice, cottonseed meal, oats, hay, barley, sorghum, cassava, and millet that are stressed by drought.

Air cell: A tiny bubble of air, created by creaming or foaming that assists in leavening dough or batter.

Ajone: A garlic extract.

Alcohol: Family name of a group of organic chemical compounds that includes methanol, ethanol, isopropyl alcohol, and others. Ethanol is produced from crops or residues with a high carbohydrate content. Alcoholic beverages contain ethanol.

Allergen: Part of a food (a protein) that stimulates the immune system of food allergic individuals. A single food can contain multiple food allergens. Carbohydrates or fats are not allergens. Most common food allergens are nuts (especially peanuts), egg, milk, histamine, etc.

Alginic acid: A polysaccharide found in seaweeds and used as thickening and binding agent in foods.

Alkali: Substance having the ability to neutralize an acid.

Alkaloid: An organic substance found in plants which is involved in the maintenance of body systems.

Allicin: A substance found in garlic, leeks and onions.

Amine: The organic base of body chemicals such as histamine.

Amino acid: Organic molecule containing both an amino group ($2NH_2$) and an acid group ; the basic building block of proteins.

Amylase: An enzyme in flour that breaks down starches into simple sugars.

Amylopectin: Highly branched-chain fraction of starch.

Amylose: Straight-chain fraction of starch.

Anaerobic: Requiring an absence of oxygen to live and grow.

Annato: A dish covered with sauce, bread crumbs or cheese and then baked or grilled and served in the same dish.

Anorexia: Eating disorder that leads to potentially fatal low body weight.

Antibiotic: Substance produced by bacteria or fungi that destroys or prevents the growth of other bacteria and fungi. Antibiotics are not effective against viruses.

Antibody: A substance produced in the blood in response to an antigen.

Antibody: A protein produced in an organism as response to the presence of an antigen (foreign body).

Antigen: A substance that can stimulate production of antibodies.

Antigen: Foreign substance (almost always a protein) that, when introduced into the body, stimulates an immune response.

Anthocyanins: Water-soluble flavonoid compounds that range in color from deep purple to orange-red.

Anthropometric: Measurement of physical characteristics of body such as height and weight.

Anticaking agent: Used to ensure the free flow in products such as dried milks, icing sugar and table salt.

Antioxidant: Substance that retards oxidative rancidity in fats by becoming oxidized itself and stopping a chain reaction.

Appetiser: A small portion of fruit, juice or savoury titbits, served as the first course of the meal.

Aroma: Distinctive, pleasant fragrance or odor.

Artificial sweeteners: Designed by man, and usually prepared by a chemical process. They are designed to supply sweetness on its own, i.e. without the carbohydrate food values which are associated with sugar. They are used by consumers who may believe it disadvantageous to use sugars for sweetening foods and drinks.

Ascorbic acid (or ascorbate): Chemical name for vitamin C. Lemon juice contains large quantities of ascorbic acid and is commonly used to prevent browning of peeled, light-colored fruits and vegetables. Green peppers, broccoli, citrus fruits, tomatoes, strawberries, and other fresh fruits and vegetables are good sources of vitamin C.

Aseptic packaging: This is a special packaging method which means that foods can last for months without refrigeration. During the process, food and packaging are sterilized by flash heating to high temperatures, killing microorganisms and pre-serving nutrients. This method is often used for milk, fruit juices and liquid egg.

Ash: Mineral content of flour; expressed as a percentage of the total weight.

Aspartame: Aspartame is a low-calorie sweetener used in a variety of foods and beverages and as a tabletop sweetener. It is about 200 times sweeter than sugar. Aspartame is made by joining two protein components, aspartic acid and pheny-lalanine.

Astringent: Shrinking or contracting of tissues in the mouth to produce a puckery effect.

Autoclave: Equipment in which high temperatures can be reached by the use of high pressure. The device is generally used for sterilization.

B

Bacteria: Large group of single-celled microorganisms which can be both harmful and helpful to food.

Barbecue: To roast slowly on a pit, over coals or under a heat unit, usually basting with a highly seasoned sauce.

Basal Metabolism: Energy used by the body, during physical, digestive and emotional rest (usually determined 12 hours after ingestion of food).

Baste: To spoon liquid over food as it cooks. The liquid may be drippings from the food itself.

Batter: A semi liquid mixture containing flour or other starch, used for production of such products as cakes and breads and for coating products to be deep fried.

Beat: To make a mixture smooth using a brisk motion that has an up-and-down movement.

Beriberi: A deficiency disease due to lack of thiamine, characterized by polyneuritis, edema, emanciation and cardiac disturbances (enlargement of heart and a very rapid heartbeat).

Betalains: Group of two types of water-soluble plant pigments: betacyanins and betaxanthins.

Beverage: Drinkable liquid that is consumed for its ability to quench thirst, for its stimulant effect, for its alcohol content, for its health value, or for enjoyment.

Biological hazard: Danger posed to food safety by the contamination of food with pathogenic micro-organisms or naturally occurring toxins.

Biological value: Measure of protein quality equal to the amount of nitrogen derived from food protein used in the body to promote growth; expressed as a ratio of the nitrogen retained to the amount of nitrogen absorbed from the food.

Biotechnology: The application of biological science to the production, modification or processing of materials. It encompasses long-established activities such as traditional plant and animal breeding, brewing, bread-making and effluent treatment, and the more modern techniques of genetic modification and the use of fermentation technology for the production of some novel protein foods.

Blanch: To apply boiling water or steam for a few minutes.

Blend: To mix two or more ingredients thoroughly.

Blood cells (corpuscles): These include red blood cells (erythrocytes) and white blood cells (leukocytes).

BMR: BMR is basal metabolic rate. Energy used by body, during physical, digestive and emotional rest (usually determined 12 hours after ingestion of food.

Boil: To cook in water at a boiling temperature.

Boiling point: Temperature at which the atmospheric pressure is equal to the vapor pressure of a liquid and an equilibrium is established.

Botulism: A food poisoning caused by the toxin produced by the *Clostridium botulinum*, an anaerobic organism, whose toxin is very powerful and only a small amount is needed to cause death.

Braise: To cook meat or poultry slowly in a covered utensil in a small amount of liquid or in steam.

Bran: The hard outer covering of kernels of wheat and other grains.

Bread: To roll in bread crumbs before cooking.

Brine: A strong solution of water and salt. Brine may also contain a sweetener such as sugar, molasses, honey, or corn syrup, for flavor and to improve browning.

Brix: A unit of measure indicating the sugar concentration of a solution.

Broil: To cook by direct exposure to radiant heat.

Broth: An unclarified thin soup.

Brown: To produce a brown surface on a food by the use of relatively high heat.

Brownian movement: The pushing to and fro of comparatively large molecules, such as those in a colloidal dispersion, by the rapidly moving small molecules of the dispersing medium (usually water in food products).

Buffer: Substance that resists change in acidity or alkalinity.

Bulimia: Eating disorder characterized by binge eating, sometimes followed by vomiting and purging.

C

Caffeic acid: An antioxidant found in many plants.

Caffeine: Caffeine is naturally found in many common foods and beverages, including coffee, tea, cola drinks and chocolate. It is a stimulant and has been proven to increase physical performance in exercise.

Calcification: Process by which an organic tissue becomes hardened by deposit of calcium salts.

Calcitonin: A hormone that is essential for healthy bones.

Calcium: Calcium is the most abundant mineral in the human body helps the body to form bones and teeth and is required for blood clotting, transmitting signals in nerve cells, and muscle contraction. Calcium helps prevent osteoporosis and play a role in lowering blood pressure.

Calorie: The amount of heat required to raise the temperature of 1 kg of water by 1°C.

Calorimeter: An instrument used for measuring the heat or energy produced (e.g. by oxidation of food).

Capillary: A small blood vessel connecting the small arteries (arterioles) and small veins (venules). Exchange of materials between the blood and tissues takes place through the walls of the capillaries.

Capsaicin: The constituent in chillies that produces a burning sensation.

Caramalization: The browning of sugar caused by heat.

Caramelize: To heat sugar until a brown color and characteristic flavor develop.

Carbohydrates: Organic compounds containing carbon, hydrogen, and oxygen; simple sugars and polymers of simple sugars.

Carcinogen: A substance that is potentially cancer-causing.

Caries: Decaying of tooth.

Carotene: A yellow-pigment found in plants.

Carotenoids: Carotenoids are natural fat-soluble pigments found in certain plants. Carotenoids provide the bright red, orange, or yellow coloration of many vegetables, serve as antioxidants, and can be a source for vitamin A activity.

Carotenoids: A group of fat-soluble, yellow orange plant pigments.

Cassava: Also called tapioca. Tropical plant with edible, starchy roots.

Catalyst: Substance that affects the rate of a chemical reaction without being used up in the reaction.

Celiac disease: The disease caused by reaction to gluten in which the lining of the intestine is damaged.

Cell: The smallest structural and functional unit of plant and mineral organisms.

Cellulose: A polysaccharide constituent of plant which passes undigested through the human digestive tract.

Chlorophyll: Green plant pigment, used for manufacture of carbohydrates from simple salts and carbon dioxide using energy derived from sunlight.

Chocolate: Any of a number of products made from fermented, roasted, grounded cocoa (or cacao) beans. Often with the addition of sugar, flavorings, and other ingredients.

Cholesterol: Vital for building hormones and cell membranes. Our body makes most of the cholesterol it needs. Cholesterol is listed under the fat information on a nutrition label. People should consume less than 300 mg of cholesterol daily.

Chop: To cut into pieces using a sharp knife or other tool.

Chymosin: Enzyme from the stomach that clots milk; previously called rennin.

Clarify: To clear a liquid of all solid particles.

Coagulation: Usually refers to a change in or denaturation of a protein that result in hardening or precipitation. Often accomplished by heat or mechanical agitation.

Co-enzyme: A helper needed by some enzymes to accomplish a biochemical change.

Coliform bacteria: Group of aerobic lactose or fermenters. Generally not harmful but their presence indicate lack of sanitation.

Collagen: The main constituent of white, fibrous tissue in the body.

Colostrum: Fluids secreted during the first week of lactation.

Colloid: Usually refers to the state of subdivision of dispersed particles; intermediate between very small particles in true solution and large particles in suspension. Proteins and pectins are usually colloidal.

Compote: Fruit stewed in syrup.

Conjunctiva: Fine membrane covering eyeball and lining of the eyelid.

Constipation: Difficulty in emptying bowels usually due to lack of water and or fiber in the diet.

Contaminated: Containing harmful substance not originally present in the food.

Controlled atmosphere packaging (CAP): Packaging method in which selected atmospheric concentrations of gases are maintained throughout storage in order to extend product shelf life. Gas may either be evacuated or introduced to achieve the desired atmosphere.

Convenience food: A manufactured product requiring a little or no preparation (other than heating, diluting or dissolving in water, where appropriate) before consumption.

Coumarins: Plant nutrients believed to help thin the blood and to help prevent cancer.

Counseling: The professional guidance of an individual in a specific area.

Cream: To mix one or more foods, usually fat and sugar, until smooth and creamy.

Cross-contamination: The transfer of harmful substances or disease-causing microorganisms to food by hands, food-contact surfaces, sponges, cloth towels and utensils that touch raw food, are not cleaned, and then touch ready-to-eat foods. Cross-contamination can also occur when raw food touches or drips onto cooked or ready-to-eat foods.

Cruciferous vegetables: A plant group that includes broccoli, cabbages, kale, cress, cauliflower, and turnips.

Crude fiber: The structural component of the plant cell wall-being the residue obtained after consecutive acid and alkali digestion of a food or food material.

Crumb: To coat or top with crumbs, such as topping a casserole dish.

Crystallization: Process of forming crystals that result from chemical elements solidifying with an orderly internal structure.

Curcumin: An antioxidant found in corn, mustard and turmeric.

Cure: A chemical agent placed in or on meat or poultry for use in preservation, flavor, or color.

Curing: Curing is the addition of salt, sodium nitrate (or saltpeter), nitrites and sometimes sugars, seasonings, phosphates and ascorbates to pork for preservation, color development and flavor enhancement.

Custard: A liquid thickened or set by the coagulation of egg protein.

Cut in: To distribute solid fat throughout dry ingredients using two knives or a pastry blender.

D

Daidzein: An isoflavone.

Dehydration: Loss of water from the body, which is not compensated by intake of water.

Dementia: Mental disorder resulting in impairment of transfer of nerve impulses.

Denaturation: Changing of a protein molecule, usually by the unfolding of the chains, to a less soluble state.

Deodorization: Removal of flavor or odor of fats during refining.

Deoxyribonucleic acid (DNA): Substance forming the genetic material in most organisms.

Dermatitis: Inflammation of skin.

Dextrinization: Breakdown of starch molecules to dextrins by dry heat.

Dextrins: Polysaccharides resulting from the partial hydrolysis of starch.

Diarrhea: Rapid movement of food matter through the digestive tract resulting in watery stools. Leads to dehydration and profound cellular disturbances.

Dice: To cut into small cubes.

Dietary fiber: In scientific terms, dietary fiber is a mixture of components derived from plant cell wall material and non-structural polysaccharides, as well as non-starch polysaccharides added to foods. It includes non-digestible polysaccharides such as cellulose, hemicelluloses, gums, pectins, mucilages and lignin. From a nutrition point of view, some authorities also include 'resistant starch' (i.e. starch that is resistant to enzymatic degradation, usually as a result of processing).

Dietetics: The feeding of the individuals according to nutrition principles.

Digestion: Mechanical and chemical breakdown of food to simple substances which can be absorbed and used by the body cells.

Diffusion: Movements of molecules from higher concentration areas to lower concentration areas.

Disaccharide: Carbohydrate made up of two simple sugars (monosaccharides) linked together. Table sugar (sucrose) is a disaccharide.

Disinfection: The application of effective chemical or physical agents or processes to a cleaned surface or to a water supply to reduce the number of microorganisms to a level consistent with good hygiene practice.

Disperse: To distribute or spread throughout some other substance.

Dispersed phase: Separated or particle component in a dispersion.

Dispersion: System composed of dispersed particles in a dispersion medium.

Dispersion medium: Continuous medium in which particles are dispersed.

Diuretic: A dietary agent that increases the flow of urine.

Dot: To place small particles at intervals on a surface, as to dot with butter.

Dredge: To sprinkle or coat with flour or other fine substance.

Duodenum: First portion of the small intestine.

E

Echinacea: A plant extract with anitviral and anti-bacterial qualities.

Edema: Accumulation of fluids in the body or parts of the body.

Edible: Intended for use as human food.

Effluent: Liquid industrial waste.

EKG: EKG is electrocardiogram. It records the electrical impulses of the heart.

Electrolytes: Essential elements essential for the cell function and for the regulation of the body fluids.

Ellagic acid: A phenolic substance found in the berries that has antioxidant properties.

Emulsifier: Surface-active agent that acts as a bridge between two immiscible liquids and allows an emulsion to form.

Emulsion: Dispersion of one liquid in another with which it is usually immiscible.

Encapsulation: Encapsulation involves the incorporation of food ingredients, enzymes, cells or other materials in small capsules.

Endogenous: Produced within the organism.

Energy: Capacity to do work. It can be manifested as heat, motion, electricity, light, etc. all of which forms are convertible into each other.

Energy density or fluence: Energy delivered from a light source per unit area ($Joules/cm^2$).

Energy metabolism: The reactions by which the body obtains and spends the energy from food.

Enriched: Enriched foods have nutrients added to them to replace those lost during food processing. B vitamins, for example, are lost when wheat is processed into white flour, so these nutrients are later added back.

Enteric: Related to the intestine.

Enzyme: Organic catalyst produced by living cells that changes the rate of a reaction without being used up in the reaction.

Enzyme technology: The study of industrial enzymes and their uses is called enzyme technology. Enzyme technology involves production, isolation, purification, and use of enzymes (in soluble or immobilized form) manufacturing of value added products in food industry.

Epidemic: A widespread occurrence of an infectious disease in a community at a particular time.

Essential amino acids: Amino acids that the body cannot make in sufficient amounts to meet physiological needs and must come from foods we consume.

Esophagus: The part of alimentary canal which connects the throat to the stomach.

Ester: Chemical combination of an alcohol and an organic acid. Fats are esters of glycerol and three fatty acids.

Equilibrium relative: Moisture content at which a food does not gain or lose weight.

Equivalence: Capability of different inspection and certification systems to meet the same objectives.

Evaporation: Loss of molecules from a liquid or solution as vapor.

Exhausting: Removal of air from within or around food and from jars and canners.

Evisceration: The removal of the viscera (internal organs, especially those in the abdominal cavity), also disembowelment.

Exchange list: A diet planning tool in which foods are organized by their nutrient and energy contents. Foods on any single list can be used interchangeably.

Excreta: Products of digestion and metabolism that is undesirable or discarded from the body in form of feces.

Extraction: Removing one material from another; Pectin is extracted from apple pomace by acid and thus made soluble.

Extraction: The technique of extraction involves movement of one or more compounds of interest (analytes) from one phase or their original location (usually referred as the sample or matrix) to another phase or physically separated location where further processing and analysis occurs.

Extrusion: Forcing a viscous solution through a spinneret-like machine (similar to a shower head). Extrusion cooking is used to produce some snack foods and breakfast cereals by pushing a dough made from a cereal flour or protein mixture into a barrel and cooking the product under pressure and at high temperature and then extruding, often causing the product to expand when it comes into contact with air.

F

Fat: Chemical unit resulting from the chemical combination or esterification of one unit of glycerine with three units of fatty acids (triglyceride). When referring to fat, under normal ambient temperatures, the product would be in solid form.

Fat-soluble vitamins: Nutrients that dissolve in fats or oils but not in water. These vitamins are often found in foods that contain fat, and fat may be necessary for their absorption from the digestive tract into the bloodstream. People who eat very little fat may have difficulty getting enough of the fat-soluble vitamins A, D, E, and K.

Farce: Any kind of stuffing.

Fatty acids: Organic acids made up of chains of carbon atoms with a carboxyl group on one end; three fatty acids combine with glycerol to make a triglyceride.

Fermentation: Transformation of organic substances into smaller molecules by the action of a microorganism; yeast ferments glucose to carbon dioxide and alcohol.

Fiber: Dietary fiber generally refers to parts of fruits, vegetables, grains, nuts, and legumes that cannot be digested by humans. Meats and dairy products do not contain fibre. Studies indicate that high-fiber diets can reduce the risks of heart disease and certain types of cancer. There are two basic types of fiber insoluble and soluble. Soluble fiber in cereals, oatmeal, beans and other foods has been found to lower blood cholesterol. Insoluble fiber in cauliflower, cabbage and other vegetables and fruits helps move foods through the stomach and intestine, thereby decreasing the risk of cancers of the colon and rectum.

Filtration: Process of passing a liquid through a filter to remove any solid particles.

Final proof: Tinned loaves are placed in a prover at 35°C (85–90% RH) until desired height is reached before baking.

Flake: To break into small pieces with a fork, being careful not to mash the pieces.

Flavanones: Type of flavonoid found in citrus fruits which provides the health benefits of neutralizing free radicals and possibly reducing the risk of cancer.

Flavor enhancers: Used to enhance or bring out the flavor and/or odor in foods without imparting a distinctive flavor of their own.

Flavors: Flavors are chemical substances added to foods in tiny amounts to ensure that food and drink tastes good and is consistent. They are obtained by chemical synthesis or isolated using chemical processes.

Flora: Bacteria occurring naturally in the intestines.

Foam: Dispersion of a gas in a liquid.

Foaming: Development and persistence of bubbles on the surface of fats during frying operations. Persistent foaming and accumulation of thick layers of foam may be indicative of fat breakdown.

Foaming agents: Used to provide a uniform dispersion of gas in a food.

Folate: One of the forms of the B vitamin folacin. Refers to the bound forms of the vitamin that are naturally present in foods.

Fold: To combine by using two motions, cutting vertically through the mixture and turning the mixture over and over.

Folic acid: Form of the B vitamin folacin in dietary supplements. It is much easier for the human body to make use of folic acid than folate.

Food: Those substances that are eaten or otherwise taken in the body to sustain psychological and physiological life; support growth and repair and replacement of tissues; and provide energy and nutrition. In essence, the sum of all the processes concerned with the growth, maintenance and repair of the body and/or its organs and systems.

Food biotechnology: Food biotechnology is the application of modern biotechnological techniques to the manufacture and processing of food.

Food-borne illness/disease: Illness resulting from acquiring a disease that is carried or transmitted to humans by food containing harmful substances.

Food-borne illness/disease/poisoning: Illnesses which result from ingestion of contaminating microbial pathogens (i.e., bacteria, mold, viruses), chemicals, parasites, viruses or from naturally occurring toxins or poisons. Bacterial foods borne disease are of two major types—intoxication and infection.

Food-borne intoxication: Illness caused by ingestion of food containing a toxin (metabolic byproduct) that was formed and excreted into the food as a result of pathogenic microbial growth (i.e. *Clostridium botulinum, Staphylococcus aureus*).

Food contamination: Foreign material that is absorbed by the food during production, processing, distribution, and food handling in the home. It includes chemical substances, such as pesticides and cleaning preparations, metals, stones, bandages, and biological materials including viruses and microorganisms causing food-borne diseases.

Food intolerance: Adverse reaction to a food or food component that does not involve the body's immune system.

Food microbiology: The study of the role that microorganisms play in food spoilage, food production, food preservation and food-borne disease.

Food processing: Using food as a raw material and changing it in some way to make a food product.

Food safety: Protecting the food supply from microbial, chemical (i.e. rancidity, browning) and physical (i.e. drying out, infestation) hazards or contamination that may occur during all stages of food production and handling-growing, harvesting, processing, transporting, preparing, distributing and storing. The goal of food safety monitoring is to keep food wholesome.

Food spoilage: Food that has decayed or decomposed. Rate of spoilage depends on surrounding environmental factors such as temperature, atmosphere and moisture. Spoiled food does not cause foodborne illness. There must be a sufficient level of hazardous material to cause such an illness.

Food waste: Food waste is a biodegradable waste discharged from various sources including food processing industries, households, and hospitality sector.

Fortification: Fortification is the process of adding nutrients to a food. Sometimes this has to be done by law, for example, in the case of margarine, and sometimes nutrients are added to help the population meet their nutrient needs, e.g. breakfast cereals.

Fortified: Addition of nutrients to food.

Free radicals: Atoms or molecules with an unpaired electron. Formation of free radicals is a normal oxidation process in foods and are formed during food treatments such as toasting, frying, freeze drying, and irradiation. They are generally very reactive, unstable structures that continuously react with substances to form stable products. Free radicals disappear by reacting with each other in the presence of liquids, such as saliva in the mouth. Consequently, their ingestion does not create any toxicological or other harmful effects.

Fry: To cook in fat. Pan-frying is to cook to doneness in a small amount of fat; deep-fat frying is to cook submerged in hot fat.

G

Galanin: A neurotransmitter in the brain that appears to play a role in the brain that appears to play a role in the desire for fat in the diet.

Garnish: To decorate.

Gel: Colloidal dispersion that shows some rigidity and keeps the shape of the container in which it has been placed.

Gelatin: A semi-solid jelly like substance or gel, used as a binding agent in salads, desserts. The dry powder is dissolved to produce the gel. Powdered fruit flavored gelatin has sugar added.

Gelatinization: Swelling and consequent thickening of starch granules when heated in water.

Genistein: A type of isoflavone that has weak oestrogen like properties.

Glace: To coat with a thin sugar syrup cooked to the cracked stage.

Glucose: A simple sugar formed by the breakdown of starch.

Gluten: Elastic, tenacious substance formed from the insoluble proteins of wheat flour during dough development.

Glycemic index: A system of ranking foods according to their effects on blood sugar levels.

Glycerol: Three-carbon organic compound (an alcohol) that combines with fatty acids to produce fats (triglycerides).

Glycogen: The form in which carbohydrate is stored in the body.

GMP: Good manufacturing practice (GMP) is that part of a food control operation aimed at ensuring that products are consistently manufactured to a specified quality appropriate to their intended use. It thus has two complementary and interacting components; the manufacturing operation itself and the control system and procedures.

Gram: Basic unit of weight in the metric system; 28.35 grams equal 1 ounce and 453.59 grams equal 1 pound.

Grind: To reduce to small particles by cutting or crushing mechanically.

Gustatory: Having to do with the sense of taste.

H

Haem iron: A form of iron found in red meats and meat products that is easily absorbed by the body.

Hazard: Any intrinsic property of a system, operation, material or situation that could, in certain circumstances, lead to an adverse consequence. In food terms, this particularly refers to an adverse consequence (health risk or loss by spoilage) to the consumer.

High density lipoprotein (HDL), a form of lipoprotein.

Helicobacter pylori: A bacterium that causes stomach ulcers.

Hemoglobin: The respiratory pigment in red blood cells that is able to bind and release oxygen.

Heparin: A acid in the liver and lungs which if injected intravenously, inhibits blood coagulation.

Homocysteine: A substance created by methionine in the body in order to repair damaged tissues.

Homogenize: To break up particles into small, uniform-size pieces. Fat in milk may be homogenized.

Hormone: A chemical secreted by endocrine glands and carried in the blood to regulate the functions of the tissues and organs.

Hydration: Process of absorbing water.

Hydrogenation: Process in which hydrogen is combined chemically with an unsaturated compound such as oil. Hydrogenation of oil produces a plastic shortening.

Hydrolysis: Chemical reaction in which a molecular linkage is broken and a molecule of water is utilized. Starch is hydrolyzed to produce glucose; water is a necessary component of the reaction.

Hydrophilic: Attracted to water.

Hygroscopic: Tending to absorb water readily.

I

Immiscible: Not capable of being mixed.

Inedible: Adulterated, uninspected, or not intended for use as human food.

Infuse: To soak a flavoring material, such as tea, leaves, herbs, bay leaf in a hot liquid in order that the liquid may absorb the flavoring.

Instant: The term is strictly justified only in the cases of dry powders or mixes which rehydrate instantly, i.e. in a matter of a few seconds (e.g. instant coffee, instant tea) and should be reserved for such speedy action. By extension, however, the term has sometimes been misused by applying it to dry mix products which rehydrate faster than some others but still take a few minutes rather than a few seconds.

Inversion: Breakdown of sucrose to its component monosaccharides, glucose and fructose.

Irradiation: Process in which food is exposed to radiant energy.

J

Jaggery: Coarse dark brown sugar made by evaporation of the sap of palm trees.

Joule: Unit of energy. One *joule* is *defined* as the amount of energy exerted when a force of one newton is applied over a displacement of one meter.

K

Ketosis: Accumulation of large quantities of ketone bodies in the body tissues or fluids this result from the incomplete oxidation of fatty acids by the liver.

Kilocalorie: Amount of heat required to raise the temperature of 1 kilogram (1,000 grams) of water 1°C; a unit of energy.

Kilogram: Metric unit of weight equivalent to a 1000 gram or 2.2. pounds.

Kinetic energy: Energy created by the very rapid movement of small molecules or ions in a liquid.

Knead: To manipulate by pressure alternated with folding and stretching, as in kneading a dough.

L

Lactalbumin: The more easily digested proteins found in milk.

Lactic acid: Three carbon acids produced in milk by bacterial fermentation of the milk sugar lactose. Lactic acid is also formed in the body during the anaerobic metabolism of carbohydrates.

Lactose: Carbohydrates found in milk, milk sugar, disaccharide composed of glucose and galactose.

Lard: To place fat on top or insert strips of fat in uncooked lean meat or fish to give flavor and prevent drying of the surface.

Leaven: To make lighter by use of a gaseous agent such as air, water vapor, or carbon dioxide.

Lecithin: Fatty substance containing two fatty acids esterified to glycerol along with phosphoric acid and a nitrogen-containing compound; a phospholipid.

Legume: Pod or fruit of peas and beans.

Lentinan: A phytonutrient found in mushrooms and thought to fight cancer.

Lethargy: State of prolong unconsciousness from which a person can be aroused but into which he immediately relapses.

Leucotriene: A substance produced by the breakdown of essential fatty acids.

Level off: To move the level edge of a knife or spatula across the top edge of a container, scraping away the excess material.

Lignin: Substance which along with cellulose, makes up the woody structure of plants. It is not a carbohydrate.

Limonoid: A flavone found in citrus fruits, especially in the seeds.

Linoleic acid: An 18-carbon unsaturated fatty acid which occurs widely in plant glycerides and is essential fatty acid needed for maintaining growth and skin health.

Lipids: Term for fats including neutral fats, oil, fatty acids, phospholipids and cholesterol.

Lukewarm: To heat at 95°C.

Lutein: A yellow-orange carotene with antioxidant effects.

Lycopene: The red antioxidant pigment present in tomatoes.

Lymph: Fluid circulating within the lymphatic system. Eventually aided to venous blood circulation, arises from tissue fluids, colorless, odorless and slightly alkaline in nature.

M

Macro: Prefix meaning large.

Maillard reaction: Browning reaction involving combination of an amino group ($2NH_2$) from a protein and an aldehyde group from a sugar, which then leads to the formation of many complex substances.

Malnutrition: An all-exclusive term of poor nourishment may result from an inadequate or excessive intake of one or more nutrients of some defect in metabolism, which prevents the body from using the nutrients properly. Inadequacy in the quality of diet or insufficient intake of one or more nutrients; may also refer to excessive intake.

Marinate: To let lie in a prepared liquid for a period for tenderizing and seasoning purposes.

Marbling: Fat distributed throughout meat.

Maturation: The process of coming to full development, maturity or adulthood.

Mayonnaise: A flavored seasoned emulsion of egg yolks and oil. Mayonnaise can be finished salad dressing or a basic dressing for other salad dressing or mother sauce for other cold sauces.

Meat: The flesh of animals used as food including the dressed flesh of cattle, swine, sheep, or goats and other edible animals, except fish, poultry, and wild game animals.

Melt: To liquefy by use of heat.

Mesophiles: Bacteria when grow at temperature between 20 and 25 °C is called mesophiles.

Micro: Prefix meaning small.

Microbiology: Microbiology is the branch of the biological sciences that deals with microorganisms, i.e. bacteria, fungi, some algae, protozoa and viruses.

Microorganisms: Very small living beings, e.g. bacteria, yeast, etc.

Millet: Small grain of Indian cereal, edible seeds of grass family which are small in size.

Mince: To divide into very small pieces by chopping or cutting.

Minerals: Inorganic substances; noncarbon compounds; ash.

Mix: To combine ingredients.

Modified atmosphere packaging (MAP): Packaging method in which a combination of gases such as oxygen, carbon dioxide and nitrogen is introduced into the package at the time of closure. The purpose is to extend shelf life of the product packaged.

Monoglyceride: Glycerol esterified to one fatty acid.

Monosaccharides: Simple sugars, for example, glucose, fructose, and galactose.

Monovalent: Having a valence of one, e.g. the valence of the hydrogen atom is 1.

Mucous membrane: A membrane lining the cavities and canals of the body that have contact with the air. It is kept moist by mucus secreted by special cells and glands.

Mycotoxins: Mycotoxin is toxic material produced by moulds.

N

Nanotechnology: Nanotechnology is a field of research and innovation concerned with building 'things'—generally, materials and devices—on the scale of atoms and molecules.

New product development (NPD): It is the process of bringing a new product to market.

Nourish: To provide food or other substances necessary for life and growth.

Nucleus: Part of the cell that contains chromosomes. It is controlled center of the cell for both chemical reactions and reproduction. It contains large quantities of DNA.

Nutraceutical: Nutraceutical = 'Nutrition' + 'Pharmaceutical'. Nutraceuticals are food or part of food which is playing a major role in maintaining normal physiological functions of the body and thus are helping in managing various health problems.

Nutrient: A substance essential for the growth, maintenance, function and reproduction of a cell or organism.

Nutritional status: Health of a person as influenced by the quality of foods eaten and the ability of body to utilize these foods to meet its needs.

O

Olfactory: Having to do with the sense of smell.

Opaque: Not reflecting or giving out light; not clear.

Organic: Pertaining to carbon compounds.

Organic acid: Contains one or more carboxyl groups (COOH). Simple examples are formic (HCOOH) and (CH_3COOH).

Osmosis: Movement of water through a semipermeable membrane from an area of low concentration of solute to an area of higher concentration to equalize the osmotic pressure created by differences in concentration.

Oxidases: Enzymes that catalyze oxidation reactions.

Oxidation: Gain in oxygen or loss of electrons.

P

Pan-broil: To cook uncovered on a hot surface, pouring off fat as it accumulates.

Panning: The cooking of a vegetable in a tightly covered skillet, using a small amount of fat but no added water.

Pare: To cut off an outside covering such as skins of vegetables.

Pasteurization: Mild heat treatment to destroy vegetative microorganisms; not complete destruction of microbes.

Pectin: Polysaccharide composed of galacturonic acid subunits, partially esterified with methyl alcohol, and capable of forming a gel.

Peel: To remove outside coverings.

pH: Expression of degree of acidity. On a scale from 1 to 14, 7 is neutral, 1 is more acidic, and 14 is more alkaline or least acidic.

pH: pH is a term used to describe the acidity or alkalinity of a solution.

Photosynthesis: Formation of carbohydrates in living plants from water and carbon dioxide by the action of sunlight on the green chlorophyll pigment of the leaves.

Phytochemicals: These are chemicals naturally occurring in plants, but are not classified as nutrients. They may have protective properties against cancers, heart disease and other chronic health conditions.

Plasticity: Ability to be molded or shaped.

Poach: To cook in a hot liquid. The food is carefully handled to retain its form as in poaching an egg.

Polyphenols: Organic compounds that include as part of their chemical structures an unsaturated ring with more than one 2OH group on it. These compounds are implicated in certain types of oxidative enzymatic browning in foods.

Polysaccharides: Complex carbohydrates containing many simple sugars (monosaccharides) linked together. Starch and pectins are polysaccharides.

Polyunsaturated fatty acid: Fatty acid that has two or more double bonds between carbon atoms. A polyunsaturated fat is one that contains a relatively high proportion of polyunsaturated fatty acids.

Pot-roast: To cook large pieces of meat by braising.

Proofing: The final rising period before baking for yeast doughs that have been molded.

Psychrophiles: Bacteria that grow at temperature less than 20°C are called psychrophiles.

Puree: To press food through a sieve or blend in blender so it becomes a smooth, thick paste. Puree can be used for soups and gravies.

R

Reduction: Gain of hydrogen or gain of electrons.

Render: To melt fat and remove from connective tissue using low heat.

Rennet: Crude extract from calf stomach containing the enzyme chymosin (previously called rennin).

Retrograde: Close association of amylose molecules in a starch gel during aging.

Retort pouch: A flexible laminated package that withstands high-temperature processing in a commercial pressure canner called a retort.

Roast: To cook, uncovered, by use of dry heat.

Roux: A thickening agent made by heating a blend of flour and fat. It may be white or brown and is used in making sauces and gravies.

S

Sachet: Herbs and spices tied in a piece of cheese cloth and added to the cooking pot or pan.

Salmonella: Genus of bacteria causing intestinal infection. Frequently contaminates foods. Salmonella is destroyed by heating.

Sanitary: Pertaining to cleanliness.

Saturated fatty acid: Fatty acid that has no double bonds between its carbon atoms and thus holds all of the hydrogen it can hold. A saturated fat is one that contains a relatively high proportion of saturated fatty acids.

Saturated solution: Solution containing all of the solute that it can dissolve at that temperature.

Saute: To cook quickly in a small amount of hot fat; a partial cooking process.

Scald: To heat milk or other liquids just below the boiling point.

Scallop: To bake with a sauce.

Scurvy: Deficiency disease caused due to lack of vitamin C in diet.

Sear: To coagulate or brown the surface of meat by the application of intense heat for a brief period.

Season: To improve the aroma and flavor of food by adding seasoning like salt, pepper, mustard, garlic.

Sewage: Refusal of liquid and solid waste (industrial or domestic waste) in sewers.

Sift: To separate the fine parts of a material from the coarse parts by use of a sieve.

Simmer: To cook in liquid at about 185°F (85°C). The liquid may show slight movement or bubbling, but the bubbles tend to form slowly and to break below the surface.

Smoke point: The temperature at which the breakdown products of fat become visible as smoke.

Sol: Pourable colloidal dispersion that has not yet set into a gel.

Solubility: Amount of a substance that will dissolve in a specified quantity of another substance.

Solute: Substance to be dissolved in another substance (called the solvent).

Solution: Mixture resulting when a solute is dissolved in a solvent.

Solvent: Substance that will dissolve another substance (called the solute).

Spore: Encapsulated, resistant form of a microorganism.

Spray drying: Spray drying is used to make liquid foods into powders by drying the liquid really quickly with hot air, making the water vaporise leaving just powder. This increases the shelf life as dry foods are less likely to be affected by microbiological spoilage. It also makes products lighter for transit. Common examples include powdered milk and egg.

Stabilizer: A substance that keeps spores, which is their resting stage. Spores are thick walled and highly resistance to heat.

Steam: To cook in direct contact with steam in a closed container. Indirect steaming may be done in the closed top of a double boiler.

Steep: To extract flavor or color at a temperature below the boiling point of water.

Sterilize: To destroy microorganisms by heating with steam or dry heat or by boiling in liquid for 20 to 30 minutes.

Sterol: An alcohol of high molecular weight, e.g. cholesterol, ergosterol, etc.

Stew: To simmer in a small to moderate quantity of liquid.

Stir: To mix food materials with a circular motion.

Substrate: Substance on which an enzyme acts or the medium on which microorganisms grow. **Supersaturated solution**: Solution that has dissolved more solute or dispersed substance than it can ordinarily hold at a particular temperature. The solution is formed by being heated and slowly cooled without disturbance.

Sweeteners: Sweeteners are additives used for sweetening foods and drink. They can either be artificial or natural and are usually many times sweeter than sugar, often with fewer or no calories. Sweeteners undergo the same strict safety testing as all other food additives.

Syndrome: A medical term meaning a group of symptoms occurring together.

Syneresis: Separation or weeping of liquid from a gel.

Synthesis: A combination of two or more substances to form a more complex substance.

T

Tactile: Having to do with the sense of touch.

Tangeretin: A flavone that may have anticancer properties.

Tannin: A substance that gives foods an astringent effect in the mouth.

Tartaric acid: An acid found in fruits, and used to flavor lemonade.

Temper: To heat fat and fry various spices before adding to a dish.

Terpene: A component of the essential oils in citrus fruits.

Thermophiles: Bacteria that grow at high temperature more than 45°C are known as thermophiles.

Thiamine: The chemical name given to vitamin B_1.

Thyroxine: It is a hormone produced by the thyroid gland which contains iodine. It helps in regulating energy metabolism.

Tissue: A collection of cells forming a structure.

Toast: To brown by means of dry heat.

Tocopherol: The synthetic form of vitamin E.

Toss: To turn food in a pan or dish by holding the container and by using a quick, jerky movement.

Toxin: A poison, usually a protein, formed by microorganisms.

Trace elements: Organic substances essential to human health and including iron, zinc and selenium.

Translucent: Shining or glowing through; partly transparent.

Trehalose: A sugar found in mushrooms.

Truss: To secure the wings and legs of a bird with pins or twine.

TVP: Textured vegetable protein that is used to stimulate meat.

Tyrosine: A non-essential amino acid made in the body and used to make dopamine and noradrenaline.

U

UHT pasteurization: Ultra heat treated or ultra high temperature pasteurization. Subjected to a relatively high heat for a defined period in order to kill microorganism and extend shelf life.

Unsaturated fat: A fat that is normally liquid at room temperature.

Urea: The final product of the deamination of amino acids.

Uric acid: An acid formed during the breakdown of nucleoproteins in body tissues and excreted in the urine.

Universal salt iodization (USI): Refers to the addition of iodine to all salt for both human and animal consumption.

Usual intake: It refers to an individual's average intake over a relatively long period of time.

V

Vasoactive amines: Amines capable of affecting constriction and dilation of veins.

Vacuum packing: Vacuum packing describes the process where the air is removed from a pack prior to sealing. This is usually to remove oxygen, resulting in extended shelf life.

Viscosity: Resistance to flow.

Vitamin: Organic compounds occurring in minute quantities in foods and essential for normal functioning of life.

Volatile: Readily forming a vapor or gaseous phase.

Volatilization: Process of becoming volatile.

W

Warm: To raise temperature to 105–114 °F.

Water activity: Water activity (aw) is a term describing the availability of water to microorganisms.

Whey: Liquid portion of milk remaining after the curd, which is chiefly the protein casein, is precipitated.

Whip: To rapidly beat such mixtures as gelatin dishes, eggs, and cream to incorporate air and increase volume.

WHO: World Health Organization of the United Nations. The specialized agency started in 1948, located in Geneva, that is concerned with health on an international level.

X

Xanthophyll: A yellow carotene with antioxidant functions.

Xerosis: Abnormal dryness on skin and eye.

Xylitol: A sugar substitute that protects against tooth decay.

Y

Yeast: Microorganism responsible for fermentation of sugars. Convert sugar into alcohol and carbon dioxide anaerobically.

Z

Zeathanxin: A carotene found in corn and egg yolk.

Zein: A protein obtained from corn and of poor nutritional value.

Zest: The colored outer portion of the peel of citrus fruits.

Zinc: A trace element needed for a healthy immune system and for reproduction.

Zingerols: A group of active ingredients found in ginger.

Zingiberene: A component of the volatile oil found in ginger.

Bibliography

1. Codex Alimentarius Commission. 2004. *Report of the 20th session of the Codex committee on general principles.* Joint FAO/WHO food standards programme. 2004 May 2–7. Paris, France. p. 44.

2. Park K, 1995. Park's Textbook of Preventive and Social Medicine, Banarsidas Bhanot Publishers, Jabalpur, 482 001.

3. Policy for a Malnutrition free Tamil Nadu. Government of Tamil Nadu, Department of Social Welfare and Nutritious Meal Programme with Technical support from UNICEF, Chennai 2003.

4. Pooja Verma. Food, Nutrition and Dietetics, 2015, CBS, Publishers and Distribution Pvt. Ltd., New Delhi.

5. Robinson Corinne H, Marilyn R Lawler, 1982. Normal and Therapeutic Nutrition Oxford and IBH Publishing Co. New Delhi.

6. Shakuntala Manay M and Shadaksharaswamy M, 1987. Foods-Facts and Principles, New Age International Pvt. Ltd., Chennai.

7. Srilakshmi B, 2003. Food Science, New Age International Pvt. Ltd., New Delhi.

8. Srilakshmi B, 2006. Dietetics, New Age International Pvt. Ltd., New Delhi.

9. Srilakshmi B, 2010. Food Science, New Age International Pvt. Ltd., New Delhi.

10. Srilakshmi, 2003, Food Science, New Age International Pvt. Ltd., Chennai. p. 171.

11. Sumati Mudambi R, Shalini Rao M, 1989. Food Science, New Age International Pvt. Ltd., Chennai.

Index